Chasing My Kudu

Or How I Ran My First Marathon

By Gerard Falotico

Chasing My Kudu
Or How I Ran My First Marathon
© 2013 by Gerard Falotico

**Cover Photo by Michael D. Ellenbogen for
Eons Creative, LLC; © 2011**

ISBN Number: 978-1-60571-184-3

SHIRES 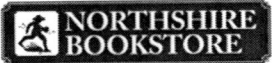 PRESS

4869 Main Street
P.O. Box 2200
Manchester Center, VT 05255
www.northshire.com

NORTHSHIRE BOOKSTORE

Building Community, One Book at a Time
*A family-owned, independent bookstore in
Manchester Ctr., VT, since 1976 and Saratoga Springs, NY since 2013.
We are committed to excellence in bookselling.
The Northshire Bookstore's mission is to serve as a resource for
information, ideas, and entertainment while honoring the needs
of customers, staff, and community.*

Printed in the United States of America

Dedicated to Jeffery Johnson, my good friend and running coach.
Without his encouragement and help,
I never would have been able to achieve my dream.

And dedicated also to my wife Anna,
without whose unwavering love and support
I would never have dared to dream the dream in the first place.

Table of Contents

"Far better it is to dare mighty things, to win glorious triumphs even though checkered by failure, than to rank with those poor spirits who neither enjoy nor suffer much because they live in the gray twilight that knows neither victory nor defeat."

—Theodore Roosevelt

Chasing My Kudu

By Gerard Falotico

PROLOGUE

The kudu, *Tragelaphus strepisceros*, is a large animal of the antelope family. It lives in eastern Africa and ranges from Ethiopia south through the Rift Valley into Namibia, Angola, and South Africa. These animals weigh 500 to 600 pounds and stand 5 feet tall at the shoulders. They vary from brown-gray to a bluish color, with white stripes on their hindquarters. Their most striking feature is the pair of exceptionally long horns that can grow up to 5 feet long. They spiral up and outward far past the ears, making almost three complete curls. The kudu is highly prized by today's hunter and safari traveler. For tens of thousands of years they served as a major food source for our African ancestors.

You may be wondering what "chasing a kudu" has to do with running a marathon. It starts like this. A few years ago, National Public Radio was broadcasting a series about how evolution shaped the human body. Each segment of the series focused on a different body part. One day it was the hand, the next day the foot, and so on. One of the topics was how and why humans became built for endurance as opposed to speed.

I was out running errands in my car when this particular segment came on. Shortly after it began, I had to stop and go into a store. By the time I returned to the car, the segment was almost over, and the reporter was ending his report with words to this effect: "So next time you are around mile 16 or 17 in the marathon and you are losing steam, think of our distant forefathers and how they would be chasing their kudus."

At that time in my life, the thought of running a marathon was only a dream in the back recesses of my mind. Still, I was interested in learning more about this "chasing kudus" stuff. So I looked up the report on the Internet. It was narrated by Christopher Joyce and aired on July 10, 2010. It delved into how humans evolved the muscles and joints needed to be long-distance runners.

We developed longer legs and smaller feet with bigger joints to absorb the pounding that occurs when we run. We also developed larger muscles, and at the same time our center of gravity shifted.

These changes occurred slowly, over millions of years. They allowed us to run down game, which provided us with the protein necessary to develop bigger brains and bodies. The prize for running for miles was a feast, which kept our forefathers and their kin fed for days. Think of it as a prehistoric barbecue. And what of those who could not run the distance? They would have had to settle for leaves and nuts and bugs.

It makes you want to run, doesn't it?

CHAPTER 1

In the Beginning

There are some things you just know in your gut. I can't say when I first realized it, but ever since my early twenties I somehow knew with absolute certainty that someday I was going to run a marathon. And don't assume I was some kind of exercise nut—far from it! I was a fat kid whose mother thought that every problem could be solved with food. When I was sixteen, I started what would be the first of many diets. I lost about sixty pounds, joined the high school wrestling team, and got in shape. Around the same time, in the early 1970s, the running craze first took off. I just wasn't interested.

I'm built more like a weightlifter than a runner. When I did track and field, I was the shot-putter. I can remember trying to run the mile in practice. I did a great first lap—and then promptly died. I simply could not do a second lap. I did get a lot of laughs, though.

Any smart person would have abandoned any thoughts of running after that, and I did for a while.

It was during my college wrestling days that I realized I could run a marathon. I was in good shape, young, strong, and optimistic. And why not? After all, everyone else seemed to be running. And there were movies like *Marathon Man* (in which, by the way, Dustin Hoffman never actually runs a marathon). But believing you can run that far, and actually doing it, are two very different things.

Fast forward to the early 1980s. I was out of school, married, with kids already and more on the way. I grew out of size 36 blue jeans to size 38. I told one of my coworkers that I had "put on a few pounds." More than a few, truth be told: from 195 to 203, and heading up. The guy grew exasperated with me. He told me, "Don't let that happen." He said that if you put on three pounds a year (which doesn't sound like a lot), after 10 years you are thirty pounds heavier. After thirty years, you are ninety pound over weight. A little math puts it all into perspective, doesn't it?

It was then that I first seriously took up running. I would wake up around dawn and run about four miles before heading off to work. It took me about a whole hour to run those four miles. That seemed like a long time. Being my worst enemy, I decided that a "good runner" would have run that distance much faster, and so maybe I should find some other exercise to do. So by the fall, when it began getting pretty dark early in the morning, I stopped. For the record, I did not find another exercise to replace it. But I remained undaunted; I still knew that one day I would run my marathon.

By the late 1980s, my weight was slowly but inexorably going up. And not just by three pounds a year, but by five. I decided to join the YMCA and give swimming a shot. Turned out I was pretty good at that. Once again, I would get up at four in the morning, go to the pool, and swim a mile before going to work. It had its benefits. Swimming kept me in good cardiovascular shape, but I still was not losing weight. Of course, I could have tried eating less. But what fun is that?

My ex-wife used to rank on me, saying that although swimming was good for my heart, I needed something more vigorous if I was serious about losing weight. She complained (and rightly so!) that I was waking up too early and therefore going to bed too early, canceling out whatever good it might be doing me. So I stopped swimming.

Some time later, and twenty pounds heavier, I decided that I really needed to try something else. It was about this time that the NordicTrack came out.

Skiing was not new to me. In fact, I had started cross-country skiing while I was in college, where I served as editor of the school newspaper. One day a flier circulating around campus fell into my hands, encouraging people to sign up for a ski touring trip to Vermont. I asked everyone what "ski touring" was. The sport was so new in America that nobody had a clue about what it might be. I figured my editorial duty demanded that I find out for myself and then write about it. So I took the trip, along with some curious classmates, car-pooling to the Viking Ski Touring Center in Vermont.

The day was cold and snowy.

Do you remember the scene in *Casablanca* when Rick reminds Ilsa about the first time they met (which was also the day the Germans marched into Paris)? He says, "The Germans wore gray, you wore blue." Well, I remember I wore blue that day too. More precisely, I wore a brand-new pair of blue jeans. For those of you too young to remember, back then the dye was not fixed in the jeans. Every time I fell (which was often!), I would leave behind a big blue spot in the snow. By the time I finished for the day, Vermont's lily-white snow was polka-dotted with blue sitzmarks.

This was also back in the days of wooden skis, which needed a vigorous waxing by hand before one ventured out onto the snow. However, I really liked the sport, so I decided to buy my own pair of skis. I must have been one of the first people to buy them, because at the time all the ski centers would let you ski free if you rented their equipment. For a while after that, the ski center operators didn't know what to do with me, because I had my own skis. So most of the time I skied free.

It had been years since I last skied; but once the NordicTrack machine came on the market, I decided to buy one in order to indulge my latest obsession. Once again, I was getting up at four in the morning to work out. And it really paid off: I finally started to lose some serious pounds. But this exercise regimen, like all the previous ones, eventually came to an end. I can't even say why this time, but I just stopped using it regularly, and then forgot about it altogether.

Guess what? The pounds came piling right back on. Are you starting to see a little pattern here? I could go on, but I think you get the picture.

CR80

Fast-forward again to the present day. I am fifty-seven years old. I finally have my feet on solid ground. The kids are grown up, and my career has been good to me. Based on what I have written so far, you might think that I am by nature capricious and irresolute in my choice of fitness regimens. However, two sports that I always liked, and stuck with, are hunting and fishing; and in my lifetime I have done my share of each. My father took me hunting as a child, and for that I remain forever grateful.

My dad was a very hardworking man. Born in Italy, he immigrated to the United States in his teens. He met my mother in New York City, where I was born in November of 1953. With only an eighth-grade education, he tried his hand at many occupations, but finally settled on being a cook. Then, when I was five months old, he bought a summer resort in Catskill, New York.

Nothing fancy, it was definitely a mom-and-pop operation. My mother served as hostess, chambermaid, baker, and whatever other role needed to be filled. My father did the cooking, maintained the property, and everything else besides. Business was mostly poor; but during the busy time, I can remember my father working until three in the morning making pizzas and running the bar. When the hotel was really full, they would have to give up their bedroom for the other help to use. My mother would sleep on a couch, while my father slept in a rocking chair on the porch.

During the winters, when the resort was closed and my father worked as a cook at one of the local restaurants, he would pass the time by reading magazines like *Outdoor Life* and *Sports Afield*. I can still remember him looking at the pictures of elk and mule deer and saying how much he wanted to go hunting for one of them. He passed away without ever fulfilling that particular dream. After he died, I swore to myself that I was not going to let that happen to me.

I did passably well in high school, but I was not the smartest kid in class by any means. When I expressed a desire to learn French, the guidance counselor suggested that I register for shop instead. He thought I was cut out more to be a carpenter than a lawyer. I would like to note that I did receive the Industrial Arts Award at graduation. After that, I had a few years of college, but then left without graduating. I still didn't know what I wanted to do for a living, so I took a job as an orderly at the local hospital; and that was only because my mother worked as a nurse's aide in the off season, and I knew it was steady work. My friends had another good laugh when I came home from work dressed in my white uniform.

One day I was given the task of shaving one of the retired doctors for his pending surgery. Watching me work, he kindly suggested that I consider becoming a full-fledged nurse and then going into the field of anesthesia. It was an excellent suggestion, as it turned out, for it gave me the incentive to finally focus on a tangible career goal. I enrolled in nursing school and later became a nurse-anesthetist. Though it was a good job, my life had the usual ups and downs, such as raising kids and getting divorced. Now I am remarried to a wonderful woman named Anna, who appreciates me and gives me the freedom to do a lot of the things that I have always wanted to do.

For a long time I charged everything on my Cabela's credit card. If you haven't heard of it, Cabela's is a big outdoor supply store. Besides selling hunting, fishing, and camping gear, they also book hunting trips. One year I saved up $3,000 worth of points and applied them toward an elk-hunting trip in New Mexico. I'm proud to say that my first time out I shot a very nice 6X6 bull elk. I think my father would have been proud too.

My wife Anna came along on that trip. While we were in New Mexico, we saw many other game animals, and Anna encouraged me to book another trip to hunt antelope and bear. The outfitter was all booked up for the following year, so we had to wait two years to make the trip. In the process of booking the hunt, the agent told me about a great mule deer hunt in Wyoming. It cost $7,000. That amount was too much to spend so soon after the elk trip, but my wife suggested that I book it two years after the antelope hunt. That would have put the hunt off for four years.

There was just one problem. I wasn't entirely sure I would be physically capable of making the trip four years down the road. You see, by this time my knees had begun to give me serious trouble. Ten years earlier I was told that I had the beginning stages of arthritis in them. Now they had gotten noticeably worse. I suffered background pain almost every day; and when I got out of bed in the morning, you could hear them pop and crack from across the room.

Not to be deterred by a little agony, a couple of Christmases ago I decided to take up racquetball again. I bought my son and me a set of racquets as presents, and off we went to the Y. I did fairly well, considering: I managed to beat my twenty-year-old son at the game.

But victory came at a cost. Both my knees became swollen; and while the right knee felt merely sore, the left one hurt like hell. It refused to bend a full 90 degrees, and I could barely walk without limping. Kneeling on it was completely out of the question. Motrin became my best friend. After about a week, the knees started to feel normal again. I celebrated by giving my son a second chance to beat me at the game. Not a wise decision! The resulting pain put an ignominious end to my racquetball phase. No big loss—I still had hunting to fall back on.

Hunting trips are ranked anywhere from 1 to 4 in the level of physically strenuous demands the sport makes on the body. Level-1 hunting (e.g., walking on level ground to a duck blind) requires very little exertion. Level-4 hunting, on the other hand, can be extremely difficult, such as when you hunt mountain goat on steep slopes at an altitude of 13,000 feet while carrying a heavy backpack and hunting gear. The aforementioned New Mexico trip was rated at 2, which is moderately strenuous.

I was told the hunt would take place at between 6,000 and 8,000 feet above sea level. We would hunt the elk by driving in a pickup truck to a good vantage point, and from there look with binoculars and spotting scopes until we found a mature bull. Then we would try stalking up close to him. In theory, it sounded simple. But as everyone knows, theory and practice are rarely the same thing.

In preparation for the hunt, once again I started showing up at the Y. I knew I had to take it easy on my knees, so I tried using the elliptical machine. This simulated the action of climbing, and I could crank up the resistance as needed. Over a few months, I got good at it, and I was able to work out for an hour at a time with the settings at moderate resistance. My weight, however, remained the big problem.

I tried the Atkins Diet, which did work up to a point. I even read the book twice. Somewhere in the middle of the book is a line that reads something like this: "At some point you may have to limit your calorie intact in order to keep losing weight." There's the rub, isn't it? As with most overweight people, limiting my calorie intake has always been the biggest challenge. I lost some weight on the diet, but it did not stay off. I'm 5' 10", and by the time I went on that hunt in New Mexico, I still weighed over 260 pounds.

Despite my weight, I thought I was at least in fairly acceptable physical shape. After all, I could do an hour on the elliptical! Our first morning out, we spotted a good bull across a big valley. I huffed and puffed a few hundred yards across the level valley floor for the stalk, but didn't take the shot. The next afternoon, we spotted some elk high on one of the ridges. We started our hike up toward the ridge. *My God*, I thought, *I wish I could die right here and now.* It would have been easier. So much for driving a pickup truck to the elk. The most embarrassing part is that I was the only one in our party having difficulties. The guide, of course, being young and fit, did fine. And though my wife (who didn't exercise at all!) was breathing heavy, she was not gasping for air the way I was. I tried to use the excuse about the air being thinner at that altitude. But that wasn't the problem. Maybe the 70 extra pounds I was carrying had something to do with it.

We eventually reached the ridge and made the stalk. I got off a good shot, and the elk went down. There was time for pictures and congratulations, and silently I told my father about what I had just accomplished.

Then the real work started. We had an 800-pound animal lying dead over a mile from the pickup truck. At least the path back was downhill all the way, but that was harder on my knees. We called for another guide to assist; and to be honest, those two did most of the work. I packed out only about 50 pounds, while the rest was carried by the guides (in two trips) or left behind to feed the scavengers. In the end, nothing went to waste.

It was then, after this hunt, that I realized that four years down the road, more than likely, I would not be physically able to go on the mule deer hunt, which was rated at a difficulty level of 3. At the rate I was going, my knees simply would not hold out. I had no idea what kind of shape my heart or blood pressure would be in by then either. After a lot of discussion with my wife, we agreed that we should just spend the money and go on the mule deer hunt the next year. I could last that long, couldn't I? And did I mention that my wife is an angel?

We paid the $3,500 nonrefundable deposit to set things into motion. I owed it to myself, my wife, the next hunting guide, and the hoped-for deer that I get into proper physical shape. I just was not sure where to begin—so I just put it off until a more convenient time presented itself. This was November of 2010. Thanksgiving was just around the corner; and after that would come the holiday parties, the seasonal treats and decorated cookies, and of course Christmas dinner. Like a seesaw, the weight went up while the motivation went down.

In February I went for my annual checkup (which I did about every five years). To start with, my doctor informed me that my blood pressure was too high, and he wanted to put me on blood pressure medication. Now, part of my job as a nurse-anesthetist is taking patients' blood pressure all day long. So if there is one thing

I know, it is blood pressure. I sporadically checked mine, and most of the time it was fair. Typically I ran high-130s to 140s over mid-80s. Well, okay, upper 80s sometimes.

It is the bottom number that one should worry about the most. This is called the diastolic blood pressure, and the top number is called the systolic. When the heart contracts, the aortic valve opens and pumps out the blood. The heart squeezes as hard as it needs to achieve adequate circulation. Even if that pressure is too high, it only stays at that level for a short period, and then the heart relaxes and the diastolic pressure drops. The subsequent relaxation of the heart muscle is responsible for the systolic pressure. The caveat here is that a healthy heart should be relaxed relatively longer than it is contracted. If during relaxation the pressure is too high, there is more time for the high pressure to damage the blood vessels that surround and nourish the heart, leading eventually to cardiac disease and a host of related problems—not least of them being death. As far as I could tell, however, my numbers were in the "safe" range, and so I was sure the doctor was wrong about my blood pressure.

He also said that he thought my blood sugar level was too high. That was an issue that *did* concern me. I have a strong family history of diabetes, and every sibling on my mother's side of the family has had the disease. Statistically, one out of four siblings born of a diabetic parent in the U.S. will contract it; and every year I look at my three brothers, and wonder which one of us it will be.

During the process of digestion, all the food we eat gets converted into glucose, which is sugar in its purest form. The glucose is absorbed by the blood and is used for energy by the cells. That is why, when your blood sugar level drops, you feel sluggish and can't concentrate. If there's no fuel, the engine can't run. However, glucose cannot move freely into the cells. In order to do that, it needs insulin, which is produced by the pancreas. If you don't have sufficient insulin to metabolize glucose, there are two basic reasons why. The first is an autoimmune issue, in which the body destroys the part of the pancreas that produces the insulin. This is what commonly happens in childhood diabetes, sometimes called Type 1.

More common among adults is Type 2, or noninsulin-dependent diabetes. It can occur when you consume too many calories, the volume of which overwhelms the pancreas. As hard as it tries, it cannot produce enough insulin to move all the sugar into the cells. Another even more common cause for this type of diabetes is age. As with so many of the other mechanisms that make up the human body, the older you get, the more the pancreas gets tired and begins to wear out. Over the years, it simply does not produce as much insulin as it once did. Either way, the symptom is the same: blood sugar levels go up. A reading of between 6 and 7 is considered diabetic. Mine was 5.9. Close, but no cigar!

At the end of the appointment, I made a deal with my doctor. For the next month I would keep checking my blood pressure, and then come back. If it really was up, I would let him prescribe something. As for the blood sugar, we decided to keep an eye on that too.

I showed up at work the next day determined to prove my doctor wrong. I got the BP machine ready, opened up a brand new cuff for myself, had a nurse wrap it around my arm, and pushed the start button. It squeezed tight and then started to deflate. I could feel the blood pumping in my arm when the machine began to reinflate, this time much tighter. It became so tight it almost hurt. How many times had my patients complained of the cuff hurting them? Maybe they were right!

Finally the cuff released and the numbers showed on the screen. I don't recall the exact reading, but the diastolic number was in the mid 90s. I thought, *This can't be right*. Frequently, the automatic machines give an abnormally high first reading, but the subsequent ones are more reliable, so I pushed the button again. This time it took its cue from the first reading and inflated really high. When it was done, the number read even higher—just over 100 diastolic. I can remember thinking that maybe I was nervous with the nurse watching me. So I put the cuff away and forgot about it.

Every morning the process repeated itself with identical results. Even when I wrapped the cuff myself, without a nurse watching, the outcome was still the same. All the readings were between 93 and 105. Even I was smart enough not to ignore this. A blood pressure that high is a heart attack or stroke just waiting to happen. So I high-tailed it right back to my doctor and got him to write me a prescription.

The first medication he put me on was in the class called ACE inhibitors. He chose this type of drug because it had the side benefit of protecting the kidneys from the damage caused by diabetes. Unfortunately, I developed the very unpleasant side effect of frequent coughing. So he changed the medication to Diovan 360 mg, the strongest dose available. I stopped coughing, and the Diovan lowered my blood pressure. My diastolic pressure was now in the mid-70s.

It was now mid-March of 2010, and I was supposed to be getting in shape for my hunt in October. So far, though, not much had happened. In fact, rather than going down, my weight had gone *up* to 280 pounds. Around that time we took a little vacation trip to Las Vegas and the Southwest. There is a photo of me standing in Death Valley wearing a white T-shirt that makes my upper torso look like a stuffed sausage. It is the kind of fashion statement where you look at the person and wonder, "What was he thinking? How could he wear something like that?" It's not as if I was happy about the way I looked. I just could not seem to muster up the motivation to do anything about it.

That was about to change.

CR&SO

On the third Sunday in April I woke up in bed alone. This was not unusual. I snored so much and so loudly that my wife could no longer sleep with me. We started off in the same bed, but almost every night she would move to the extra bedroom. The snoring had gotten so bad that the cats would move out too. But this morning, something was different.

Upon waking, I immediately noticed a funny feeling in my chest. The best way to describe it is that it felt like butterflies fluttering around my heart. Believe me, this is a lot less pleasant than it sounds! As a trained anesthetist, I knew instantly what was happening to me: my heart had gone into atrial fibrillation. I just wouldn't believe it. I lay there thinking, *Shit, this can't be real.*

At first I tried to convince myself that maybe it was just a very fast heart rate. This had happened to me years ago. Every now and then my heart would start racing to around 150 beats per minute, but then slow back down. My doctor told me at the time that it was SVT, or supraventricular tachycardia. He suggested that I cut out the caffeine; and afterward, I never had the problem again.

No, what was happening to me now was not a relatively benign tachycardia. This was most definitely atrial fibrillation, a type of cardiac arrhythmia (irregular heart beat) that can lead to congestive heart failure or stroke. I tried all the usual noninvasive, first-resort maneuvers we in the medical field try in order to break this kind of irregular heart rhythm, such as applying pressure on the eyes and messaging the carotid artery. None of these worked. I even tried thumping on my own chest, a technique known in some medical circles as a "2-joule deliberation." I have never actually heard of this working—but hey, what did I have to lose?

A little knowledge is a dangerous thing, as they say. If this were my patient, I would have taken immediate action. If it were a friend or family member, I would have insisted on their going straight to the hospital. Oh, but not me! Instead, I went downstairs and watched television. I didn't feel that bad, after all. There was no chest pain, and I was neither lightheaded nor short of breath. My hope was that the episode would end spontaneously before my wife got up.

It did not.

When she woke up, I had to tell her what was going on. Of course, she wanted me to go right to the hospital. My first instinct was to hem and haw and drag my feet. Anna would have none of it. She may be a petite lady—but boy, is she tough! She knows just how to get things done. She said that if I didn't get into the car immediately, she was going to call my kids, wake them up (after what was most likely a busy night of drinking and partying), and let *them* deal with me. I knew I could not win this battle. One way or another, I was going to the hospital, so I agreed to go—as long as I could drive myself. If I had to go seek medical attention against my will, at least it would be on my own terms.

The only good thing about this situation was that it occurred on early Sunday morning, and so there was no one else in the emergency room. After we arrived, things happened quickly. We told the triage nurse what was going on, and right away she performed an initial ECG. It showed exactly what I first suspected: A-fib with a heart rate of 140. I wasn't going anywhere. They put me into an examination room, where little spots of my chest hair were shaved off for the ECG stickers, an IV was started, and someone took an X-ray of my chest. The main thought that ran through my head was: *So this is what it is like to be a patient.*

When the doctor arrived, he took my history and did a physical. Afterward, we discussed my options. He first wanted to try giving me medication to slow the heart rate, with the hope that I would convert to a normal rhythm. I agreed. He had the nurse administer 20 mg of metoprolol to me intravenously in 5 mg dosages. It did slow my heart rate to 120, but the A-fib continued.

The treatment of atrial fibrillation can be complex and varies widely, depending on the severity of the symptoms and the patient's overall condition. I knew that if they did not fix my rhythm soon, then they would have to put me on blood thinners for several weeks or months. They might try other medications; and if none of those worked, the last resort would be cardiac defibrillation (where they use a set of paddles to give the heart an electric shock as a means of restoring normal rhythm). I also knew that the longer I was in A-fib, the harder it would be to fix.

Since we knew the time that it had started (sometime between 3:30 A.M., when I woke up for a few minutes, and 5:30 A.M., when I got out of bed), the cardiologist recommended that we try defibrillating me sooner rather than later. This procedure is almost 100% successful within the first few hours of the onset of A-fib, but the experience can be somewhat unpleasant. I didn't really want to go that route, but I did want to get better. Because my choices were limited, and I was running out of time, I reluctantly agreed to the cardiac defibrillation. I thought, *Hell, this is what I do to other people; it's not supposed to happen to me!*

There are several reasons why you would defibrillate someone. The first and most critical reason is that the person's heart has gone into a life-threatening rhythm that needs to be addressed "stat." This is what you see in the movies and TV shows when they call "code blue" and everyone comes running. At that point the patient is unconscious and does not need sedation before being shocked. Another reason is that the patient's rhythm is normal, but the heart is beating too fast. A third reason is that the rhythm is abnormal but is not immediately life-threatening, as in the case of A-fib. With the latter two conditions, the patient is conscious and thus would be aware of getting shocked.

Nowadays, medical practitioners rarely use the kind of paddles that you see in the movies, which are pressed and held directly onto the chest. Instead, they apply a pair of pre-gelled adhesive pads onto the back, one between the right shoulder and spine and the other on the left side just under the armpit. These new pads ensure an even spread of the conductive jelly, which allows for a more uniform application of the shock. Simply put, there is less chance of getting burned from the electricity (although the area under the pads frequently looks and feels like it has sunburn).

The shock itself would hurt if you were not sedated, but it is so brief in duration that most people wouldn't classify it as horrible pain. What is most unpleasant is the way the patient jumps when he or she is shocked. This reaction is totally involuntary and is not the result of the pain. It happens because the electrical energy that resets the heart also causes the other muscles to contract. In the movies, patients are depicted as leaping into the air when shocked. In reality, the arms frequently rise up and the legs twitch a bit, but that is all.

It is very rare to shock someone without sedation first—especially when that someone is himself an anesthetist, not to mention the world's biggest wimp. There was *no way* that anyone was getting near me with 200 joules of electricity while I was awake!

On occasion, the cardiologist will administer a heavy tranquilizer for sedation; but most of the time, an anesthesia provider is called. They have much better drugs—the kind that can render you unconscious within seconds and lasts for only a couple of minutes. They are also the experts in airway management. If there is a breathing problem, they can assist with oxygen intake until the patient wakes up.

Almost as soon as I made the decision to go ahead with the cardioversion, I heard a series of overhead pages, the meaning of which would have been a mystery to non-medical personnel. But because this is my turf, I knew what was going on. Somewhere there was a mother in labor whose baby was suffering some type of fetal distress. One of the pages announced, "Anesthesia to Labor and Delivery stat." Shortly after that they called a Code C (stat emergency, get the baby out right away by caesarean section). The personnel attending my case would likely be busy elsewhere for a while, so nothing was going to happen to me any time soon. I was actually relieved, but knew the reprieve would not last forever.

As reprieves go, I've had better. In a way, having the "luxury" of time to think about what is to come can be worse than the procedure itself. No one who has not experienced it first-hand can imagine the feelings of helplessness and vulnerability that assail the mind as one lies alone on a hospital bed, hooked up to tubes and machines. You hope against hope that the people who are supposed to take care of you know what the hell they are doing. At a time like this, even the most optimistically inclined patient cannot help but contemplate worst-case scenarios. What if the procedure doesn't work? What if there are "complications"? *What if I die?*

It was a good hour and a half before the medical team finally got back to me. First the nurse wheeled in a resuscitation cart. It had all the medications needed in the unlikely event that my heart stopped. I say "unlikely," but I was not feeling lucky that day. Then they brought in the defibrillator, laid out the rest of their equipment, and told me that the anesthesiologist would arrive shortly.

My palms and armpits began to sweat profusely. When the anesthesiologist did arrive, he was carrying a large syringe filled with a milky-looking substance. I recognized what that substance was immediately: it was Diprivan, generically known as propofol (which may be more familiar to readers as the drug that killed Michael Jackson). I knew it well, as I myself used it on almost every patient every day.

We made a little small talk, and then we got down to business. He asked me the pertinent questions, looked at my lab work, glanced at the ECG monitor again, and then announced, "Let's get started." I gave my wife a kiss (hopefully in "farewell" and not as "goodbye"!), and she headed off to the waiting room.

The nurse opened my gown to apply the pads. One look at my chest stopped her in her tracks. She said that my chest was too hairy; she would have to shave it. I hate that. Several years before, I had undergone a stress test, and at the time they shaved the spots to put on the ECG stickers. That entire summer my chest looked ridiculous: black hair with big white spots. I don't mean to be vain, but I thought, *At least now the hair is all gray; maybe it won't be so noticeable this time.* The nurse left to get a razor. When she returned, I noticed she held a large dollop of shaving cream in her left hand. It reminded me of fresh whipped cream, and I couldn't help but think how good that would taste.

Before the nurse could begin shaving me, the anesthesiologist took another look at the monitor and said, out of the blue, "Look, he converted." Sure enough, my heart rhythm had returned to normal. Saved by the bell! Or rather, saved by my hairy chest. The unexpected need to shave me had provided just enough of a delay for my heart to convert all by itself. Otherwise, I would have been unconscious and shocked into rhythm by now. My first reaction was to look at my heart rate to make sure the medication they had given me earlier had not slowed my heart rate too much, but all was well. They called in the cardiologist and told him what had happened. He looked disappointed, but had little choice but to give me a clean bill of health.

As for me, I packed my bags and ran.

CHAPTER 2

A New Direction

Talk about a reality check. No matter where I went from here, life would never be the same. Either I had to change my lifestyle or I would begin a gradual but inexorable decline toward an inevitable and miserable end.

No one plans on getting fat, growing old, and losing the ability to do the things one wants to do—and once used to do with ease. All too often it happens anyway, mainly because we let it. Big life changes tend to occur by imperceptible degrees, and thus we learn to accept them over time, because they don't seem so big at the present moment. Then one day you wake up, look back, and are stunned by the enormity of the change, and realize that now you can't do anything about it. You may want to, you may yearn for it. But it is too late. Maybe your hips hurt too much. Maybe you get too short of breath. Or maybe you are too beaten down from years of failure to muster the energy to change. And so you throw in the towel, sitting weary and bloodied in your corner of the ring, waiting for the Referee to ring the last bell of the last round of the fight of your life.

Following this frightening episode in the hospital, that's where I stood in my mind: teetering precariously on the edge of the crevasse that separates us from the Great Beyond. One more disappointment, one more *I can't*, one more *I don't give a damn*, and I would spiral down a path from which no one returns, and the only outcome of which is a premature death from some serious but treatable medical condition that could have—and should have—been all too easily avoided, if one only had the will.

I went on the Internet in search of a healthy diet. I was hoping to find something that advised a normal portion size, and how much of each food group I needed. In the past, if I were allowed two servings of pasta, I would load my plate full. Then I could have a second serving, equally full on the plate. And it wasn't a small plate either!

I think every newspaper in the country should publish a full-page ad, three times a week, depicting the food pyramid and suggesting how many calories the average person requires every day, as well as the number of calories contained in single servings of different types of food. The government should pay for this.

Considering the billions this country spends on health care every year because of poor diet, this strategy would save money in the end. I am an intelligent and motivated man who knows how to use the Web for research, and I was having a hard time finding what I needed to know. Imagine if you were *not* motivated. You would never locate a source of correct, consistent information.

One of my thoughts was to see a nutritionist and have a professional get me started on a proper dietary regimen. I called one up to make an appointment and was immediately scheduled in, but was advised to talk with my insurance company first to confirm that they would cover the service. To my surprise, Blue Cross informed me that my plan would not cover visits to a nutritionist unless I was a diabetic. I explained to them that I had been diagnosed with metabolic syndrome and was probably pre-diabetic. In so many words, their response was: "Sorry Charlie. If you don't have full-blown diabetes, we are not paying."

This makes absolutely no sense to me. Treating a chronic condition such as diabetes would cost the insurance company an extraordinary amount of money over the years, compared to the relative pittance required to provide me with the tools to prevent it in the first place. Again, think of the savings if the government mandated this coverage. It would pay for itself many times over. But there is no such mandate, and Blue Cross has its rules. So it seemed that if I wanted to see a nutritionist, I would be paying out of pocket. I had little choice but to make the appointment, and hope it didn't cost an arm and a leg.

Remember, I had planned and paid for a deer-hunting trip out west, coming up in just a few months, which I knew would involve some serious climbing. To physically prepare for this expedition, my wife and I decided that we (meaning "I") needed to do more hiking in addition to the gym exercises I intended to start soon. It was almost spring; and with the nicer weather, we wanted to get outdoors anyway. There is a little mountain close to our home called Hadley Mountain. The trail to the summit provides the kind of moderately difficult day-hike that the Boy Scouts would do. A lot of people climb it to get warmed up for the summer hiking season. Though I have lived near the mountain for twenty years, I had never tried to climb it. Now I wanted to give it a shot, not just for fun and fitness, but mostly because an acquaintance of mine with whom I have a bit of a contentious relationship had climbed it the summer before. He is older than I am and has bad knees. If Arden could do it, then I could do it.

We started out one Sunday afternoon, thinking we had plenty of time to tackle the ascent and get back before nightfall. After all, it has an elevation gain of only about 1,500 feet. While driving toward the mountain, we passed a restaurant that we knew served decent food. One needs energy to climb, right? So we decided to stop for a pre-hike bite to eat. I can't remember what my main dish was—maybe chicken, maybe salmon. But whatever I had ordered, it included grilled vegetables. You know—*healthy* food? And boy, did they hit the spot!

Some things happen for a reason. Little did I realize then that those vegetables would become a staple for me.

After our late lunch, we drove to the trailhead and parked. I laced on my boots and got out the hiking sticks. I had made them myself years before, cutting a couple of maple saplings—one to about six feet for me and the other a little shorter for Anna—and then lopping off the branches with a hatchet and smoothing down the nubs. Mine had a small depression where one of the nubs did not cut out clean. It was in just the right place, so that when I walked and swung the stick in front of me, my thumb rode in and out of the groove. I had also drilled a hole at the top and strung in a loop of rawhide shoelace, the purpose of which was more decorative than functional.

In retrospect, we had started the hike later in the afternoon than we should have. We only had about two and a half hours of daylight left, which initially I figured was more than enough. Forty-five minutes up and a half hour down was my best estimate. Signing into the trailhead book, we began to walk. The first few hundred yards were a piece of cake. Shortly after, however, I broke into a sweat and started to huff and puff. *You just need to warm up and find your stride*, I told myself. Soon the sweat began to soak through my shirt, but still we continued up.

Eventually we hit an area of smooth basalt rock (which forms the foundation of the Adirondack Mountains) where the trail becomes much steeper. More than once I had to stop and catch my breath. This was supposed to be easy—after all, Arden had managed it! Anna was doing fine and kept asking me if I wanted to turn back. I was not sure how I would finish the climb, but I was determined to keep going. I wondered, though, if we had enough daylight left (and, secretly, hoped that we did not).

After about one more hour of tortured climbing, we met another hiker on his way down. He told us that the section just ahead was the last bad leg of the trail, and then it would level off. He also mentioned that the trail was almost two miles long from top to bottom. *What?* I had been expecting a hike of 1,500 feet, not two miles!

Our informant was right: the next section *was* a killer. After that, though, the trail did level off. At last, the fire tower at the summit came into view. We had made it! Sure, it had been hard, but the panoramic view made it worth the effort. Nearby we could see Great Sacandaga Lake and, in the distance, the High Peaks of the

Adirondacks. By now the sun was heading quickly toward the western horizon, and after a few pictures we headed back down. I should have been proud of my accomplishment and exhilarated by the physical effort. Instead, I felt embarrassed about what poor shape I was in. And everything hurt: my knees, my legs and, most of all, my ego.

With gravity on my side, the descent seemed easier—but not by much. Somewhere around halfway down we stopped and rested and made small talk. I mentioned to Anna that for years Arden and I had wanted to hike to Lake Tear of the Clouds on Mount Marcy, which forms the headwaters of the Hudson River. It is at least a 16-mile hike, and I didn't think I would ever get to do it. Some people would have said, "That's too bad." Others would have said, "You should have done it when you were younger." Still others would have said, "You should have never let yourself get so fat." Anna, bless her heart, said none of those things. Instead, she proclaimed, "Let's make that our goal for the summer." It was then and there that I decided to start working on some of the things on my bucket list—and right at the top was the hike to Lake Tear of the Clouds.

Was that a kudu I just heard rustling in the bushes?

03&80

My appointment with the nutritionist was scheduled for May 15. I had no idea what to expect. I hoped against hope that she might offer some quick fix or magic weight-loss potion that would get me started, but I knew there was slim chance of that happening. So I felt none too optimistic when I entered her office.

Shannon was a very pleasant lady with a small frame and red hair. The top of her desk was covered with nutrition books, academic journals, and realistic plastic models of different foods scaled to healthy (meaning "small") portion sizes. I told her my story, complete with all the usual rationalizations, excuses, and broken self-promises. It was a tale I'm sure she had heard a million times before. I felt a little bad for her. Surely she did this same dance with all her patients. After all, who were her patients? Very likely, they were mostly older people who had spent a lifetime developing poor eating habits, with the inevitable health results— and now they expected her to turn things around with the snap of her fingers. That described me to a T. I thought of my food-loving Italian grandmother. Would she walk into that office and expect to come out with a completely different approach to eating? Hell would freeze over first!

In the middle of our conversation I received a text on my iPhone, which I had rudely forgotten to turn off. Watching me hastily power it down, she mentioned that there was an app available called *Lose It!*, which I could download for free. Then she weighed me (280 pounds!), we scheduled another appointment, and I left. This was my last hope, and nothing had come of it—no miraculous pill, no foolproof diet, no magic words to inspire a major lifestyle change. Heading home, I felt completely defeated. Little did I realize that she had opened the door to a whole new world for me. I just didn't know it yet.

At home, I told my wife about the visit. Anna offered to download the app for me, which I had no desire at all to do for myself, given my state of discouragement. As it turned out, the app was very well designed and easy to use. One simply enters pertinent information, such as height, age, current weight, and weight-loss goals. Then it calculates how many calories the user can consume each day in order to reach those goals over a specific span of time.

I thought, *Maybe there is such a thing as magic after all!* To work its magic, the app relies on an extensive database of foods and the calories they contain. In addition to listing many supermarket foods, this database includes the menus of most fast-food restaurants, and their calorie counts as well. Want to know how many calories in a Panera's turkey sandwich or a Papa John's pizza? *Lose It!* will tell you. Curious to compare Kraft Macaroni & Cheese dinner with Kashi Honey Sunrise cereal? The app has this information too at its virtual fingertips. It can tell you how many calories are contained in ground beef as compared to ground turkey, and for just about anything else that's edible. Once you know what you want to eat and what it will cost you in calories for a specific portion, you can look up how many calories are burned by doing different exercises, whether it's swimming or tennis or even vacuuming.

After every meal and snack, you enter the quantity consumed. Next, you enter the type of exercises you did that day, and for how long. Finally, through simple arithmetic, it tallies up the net gain (or loss) of calories consumed that day. One of the best features of the app is the simple visual reinforcement that it provides. A bar graph keeps track of your calorie intake and exercise regimen. When you eat (or consume calories), the bar moves to the right. When you work out (or burn off calories), it moves to the left. If you pass your pre-set calorie limit for the day, the bar turns from green to red to alert you that you need to cut back on the food or exercise some more. Besides keeping a record of your daily calorie count, it also lets you monitor your progress across weeks and months. These results can be emailed to anyone you choose. I sent mine to Shannon, the nutritionist, so she would know how I was doing and that I was serious about taking control of my weight and diet.

Of course, this app only works if one is 100% honest and absolutely faithful about recording everything pertinent to taking off one's excess weight. I told all my friends about *Lose It!*, and several have tried it. The one thing I stressed to them is that simply having the app on your phone will not magically cause you to lose weight. You need to adhere to the program. I had one friend show me his progress bar, and 3 out of 7 days during the week he had crossed into the red zone. His excuse? "It's summer, I want to barbeque and drink beer!" In other words, his philosophy was *Eat, drink, and be merry.* Okay, I get that. It is damn difficult to deprive oneself of epicurean pleasures. After all, you only live once. But the key word here is "live." Once you're dead, you don't get to enjoy those pleasures at all. Better to pace yourself and enjoy them in moderation—for a long time. The trick behind making this app work, then, is that the desire to be thinner must be stronger than the desire to overeat.

For that reason, I set for myself the modest but doable goal of losing two pounds per week, so I would not be tempted to cheat. In the beginning, the app kindly gave me plenty of calories to live on—over 2,100 to start! I had to choose my food wisely, and in smaller portions than I was used to, but I could still eat a lot. Nevertheless, limiting my calorie intake this way was harder than expected, causing me to act awfully crabby for the first few weeks.

The good news is—it worked! I can't say for sure why this app was so effective in my case. Maybe it was the visual feedback, or maybe it was the inherent discipline that a mathematical approach imposes on the mind. Whatever the case, whenever people asked me why it worked so well for me, I would just say, "I'm hungry—hungry to lose weight."

CRSO

I clung to this app religiously month after month. Only once did the progress graph slip over into the red zone, and that was during a weekend when we had company. An old friend of my Russian-born wife came to visit from abroad, and that's what did me in. I should have guessed what was coming the minute the doorbell rang. When I opened the door, a man I'd never met before stepped in and handed me a bottle of vodka. The first words out of his mouth were: "Stick this in the freezer so we can start drinking it." I tried to behave myself; but anyone who has spent any social time with Russians knows that they love to eat and drink—and they refuse to do it alone. Despite my best intentions, that weekend visit with Anna's friend turned into two solid days of overindulgence and general merrymaking. Red zone or not, I'm only human.

Those two "off-the-wagon" days aside, I managed to lose four pounds each of the first two weeks, then leveled off to a couple of pounds a week. Some weeks, the readout on the bathroom scale did not change much, which was a disappointment. Then other weeks I'd see a big drop, and that's what kept me going.

Soon my weight was down by about 15 pounds, at which point I decided I was ready for our next hike. This time we planned on tackling Prospect Mountain, at the southern end of Lake George. It had been years since I last climbed it, around when my youngest son was 3 years old. I remember carrying him on my shoulders for several hundred yards at a time. How hard could it be? Having shed so many pounds in the past few months, I expected this hike to be a breeze. Wrong again! What a bitch of a climb. Just like my last outing, I thought the exertion was going to kill me. No doubt about it: I had a long way to go still before I dared attempt the more than 16-mile trip to Lake Tear of the Clouds. But I refused to give up.

Our goal was to hike to the lake by summer's end. They call it a "lake," but it is more like a nondescript pond on the far side of Mount Marcy, the tallest mountain in New York State. Believe it or not, this glorified puddle is the source of the mighty Hudson River. Born of the runoff from the surrounding mountains, Lake Tear of the Clouds is surrounded by marshy flats where the water collects and then fills the pond. From here the Hudson begins its 150-mile journey, spilling out in a small stream that runs over a bed of rocks rounded smooth by thousands of years of erosion. Standing on the shore, you can look north and see Mount Marcy towering above you.

The shortest direct hike to the lake is 11 miles in length over tough trails. Or you can take a shortcut and climb Mount Marcy, passing by the lake along the way. If you chose that route, it is only an 8-mile hike each way. I cannot say for sure why I have always wanted to hike there. Perhaps it is the remoteness of the lake—the romance of standing in a place that not many people will ever visit. Or maybe it is the interesting historical fact that Teddy Roosevelt was camping there when he got word that President McKinley had been shot. He made the trek back out in the dark. Whatever the reason, every time I drive over the Tappan Zee Bridge, I look to the north and feel an irresistible urge to see the modest birthplace of this mighty river.

During the course of the summer, we made several more hikes, each longer than the last. The most memorable one was near the Cedar River, where I managed to get lost on a circular trail for hours—not exactly my proudest moment as a woodsman! What I *was* feeling proud about was that by this time I had dropped over 30 pounds, and now I was on my third pair of smaller-sized pants. I could see the difference in myself, and so could Anna. But no one else seemed to notice. I attributed this to the fact that I still looked like a sausage (just not quite as stuffed as before). The thing that really got my goat was that around this time one of my coworkers, who was also using the app, had lost the same amount of weight. The only difference is that he had less to lose, and so he started from a lower point. As a result, his weight loss showed more. Everyone would tell him, "You look so good, you've lost so much weight!" Then I'd pipe up, "Hey, what about me? I lost just as many pounds as he did." They would look at me in disbelief and say, "Really? Oh, then you look good too." I found this frustrating—but a little funny too.

⊗⊗

Summer was nearing its end, and the days were getting shorter, the nights cooler. We decided to take one more hike in the Mount Marcy area to get familiarized with the terrain. This was a smart move. We realized that we could not travel deep into the High Peaks and then take such a long hike, all in single day. We would need to drive up the day before and stay overnight. That way we could tackle the trail first thing in the morning, fresh and rested. We scheduled our hike for the first weekend after Labor Day.

By this time my weight was dropping fast. I found myself buying a new pair of pants every two weeks. I was pleased as punch with my progress, of course; but investing in a new wardrobe twice a month was starting to get expensive. This is a problem I wish on all my overweight friends! To save money, I ended up buying the cheapest jeans I could find. I was down about 60 pounds—and now *everyone* was noticing.

At last the weekend of our hike arrived. We drove to Lake Placid and spent the night in a hotel. Even though it was still fall, we awoke the next morning to below-freezing temperatures. Still, the leaves were near their peak, and the mountains had become a kaleidoscope of bright reds and yellows and oranges. What a great day to spend in the woods! We hit the trail at first light, around 6:00 A.M.

As mentioned earlier, there are two ways to get to Lake Tear of the Clouds: climb to the top of Mount Marcy and go down the other side (seven miles up and another mile down); or take the long trail around (11 miles). Although the latter route meanders between the big mountains, it still involves a lot of uphill walking. That was the way we chose.

The first 2½ miles were relatively easy. This got us as far as Marcy Dam, a small wooden structure that would be washed away a year later by Hurricane Irene and Tropical Storm Lee. From there we continued along a crystal-clear brook. In years gone by, it held brook trout, but acid rain has killed them all. We crossed over the brook and took the left-hand trail toward Lake Arnold. Here things began to get tough, with lots of uphill walking, and clambering from rock to rock. I was glad we had the hiking sticks.

Lake Arnold turned out to be a very pleasant surprise. For one thing, it's more of a pond than a lake. What is interesting is that you actually walk up to it from below water level. As you approach the beaver dam, which makes up one edge of the pond, you find yourself eyeball to eyeball with the water's surface. Crowning the pond on the far side is Mount Colden, the eleventh highest mountain peak in New York. The view is very pretty, and worth every step we took to get there. After a short rest, we were on the move again.

We continued up—then continued down—and then made our way through some marshy terrain. We were deep into the Adirondacks now. It was a smart idea to do this hike in the fall. During spring or summer, one is sure to be eaten alive by black flies and mosquitoes. We finally arrived at a fork in the trail that would lead us to our goal. We were only a mile away now. We rested a bit, then continued toward the end of our journey. It involved yet more uphill climbing, of course. Lake Tear of the Cloud would not give herself up easily.

At 11:30 in the morning we crested the last rise, and beheld the object of our quest: a small, shallow, mud-filled puddle lined with marsh grass. Yet after our exertions, it seemed the most beautiful sight in the world, something that I had dreamed of seeing for years. We stood there for a while, just staring at it, not sure what to do. When you want something so badly, and then work so hard to achieve it, reaching the goal at last seems almost anticlimactic. As with most things in life, it is not the destination that matters, but rather the journey. This particular journey was 35 years old, many dreams long, and it cost me 60 pounds of superfluous fat. It was also the first thing I managed to check off my bucket list. I thought of myself lying on that stretcher in the emergency room just months earlier, looking down at my big belly, and thinking I would never see Lake Tear of the Clouds. Hah! Never say never.

We took some pictures, ate lunch, relaxed, and then took some more pictures. After all the effort I had made to get here, I was reluctant to leave. But I had to keep in mind that we were deep in the woods and had to get back before dark. The original plan was to return the way we had come. The hike had been far from boring; but now I was primed to see something new. Overhead loomed the back side of Mount Marcy, the alternative route back our car. The summit looked very high and very far away. But that route was also shorter. So that's the way we decided to go. We packed up our things, took a few more pictures, and then started up.

Much to my surprise, the first part of the climb was less chal-lenging than I had expected. About halfway up the mountain, however, the trail became rather steep. Here we had to use our legs and hands, clambering from rock to rock and tree to tree. Once we passed the tree line, though, we had nothing to grab onto. A good portion of the climb was at a 30-degree angle, and I am pretty sure some parts were 45 degrees. Nevertheless, I was thankful to be going up rather than down. Some of the hikers we passed along the way traveling in the opposite direction were having a hard time of it. With no trees around to grab for balance, they often slid down the trail many feet at a time. If they got up a good head of steam, they might end up reaching the bottom ass over teakettle. It looked pretty unsafe to me.

Eventually we made it to the cold, windy summit of Mount Marcy. We were tired and sweaty; but from here we could glance down at the little pond from where we had started. I was very satisfied and pleased with myself. By dint of hard work and lots of support, I had accomplished something that I always wanted to do but thought I never would.

Now the trail home lay before me, seven miles long—but at least it was all downhill!

We got out of the woods at 6:00 P.M., just as it was getting dark. When we told the forest rangers where we had been, they could hardly believe that we had done it in one day. For someone my age, that was practically unheard of.

ᏬᏒᎩᎾ

Clearly, dropping 60 pounds of fat was a big factor in the successful completion of this hike. I was still losing weight, but not as fast as before. My original goal had been to lose 80 pounds. Now that I was so close to my goal, I decided to shoot for 85, which would put me below 200 pounds. I had not seen those numbers on the scale since the time I was in anesthesia school over thirty years ago.

Now, with less weight to carry around, my knees were feeling better. When I got out of bed in the morning, they still snapped and popped, but the nagging pain was gone. I can't say when it happened exactly; but one day I realized that they had stopped hurting. What a sea change. Hadn't I just spent a ton of extra money on my upcoming hunting trip, reasoning that in another two years I wouldn't be able to walk uphill because my knees would hurt so much? Now look at me—climbing entire mountains without any pain at all!

It was around this time, with the recently shortened bucket list fresh on my mind, that I had the first remote thoughts of running a marathon. Up until now I believed that such a goal was simply beyond my physical reach. But what's the harm in dreaming? Little did I know that the dream would soon become an obsession. I certainly could not tell people about it. Everyone would look at me and laugh—everyone, that is, except for my friend Jeff.

I was working out three to four days a week, mostly on the elliptical machine at the Y. Some days I swam for an hour without stopping. My endurance was way up, and my weight continued to drop. By the beginning of October, there was not one minute of my daydreaming time that I did not spend thinking about running a marathon. When I say "not one minute," I mean that quite literally. The thought of it consumed all my waking hours, and probably some of my sleeping ones too.

Call it luck, call it fate, or call it divine intervention. Whatever you want to call it, some things just happen for a reason. And the thing that happened was that somebody told me about a website called Woot.com. It offers one product a day at a much-discounted price. Every day I would visit the site, but I never saw anything I really wanted. Then one morning, while visiting the site as usual, I saw a treadmill for sale. My first reaction was: "I don't need that."

But for some reason, a voice in my head kept telling me to look at it again.

I thought, *If you get it, are you really going to use it?* Not likely. Even with the discount, the price was anything but cheap. Would this become just another expensive toy that ended up being used as a clothes rack? I talked with my wife about it. She was somewhat interested, but I still wasn't sure. I argued with my inner voice. *What if I never run a marathon?* To which my inner voice replied, *What about those cold winter mornings when you don't feel like venturing out to the Y?* The more I thought about it, the better I liked it. Anna felt the same way too. It really wouldn't be a wasted investment if she used it as well. By mid-afternoon, we both decided it was worth buying the treadmill. Even if neither of us used it, what would be the loss? You can never have enough clothes racks, right?

We already had the perfect spot picked out for it. The previous owners of our house had added an extra three-season room, which we converted for year-round use by insulating and heating it. The room, done in knotty pine with large windows and skylights, is bright and cheery and overlooks the small pond and bird feeders in our back yard. This is where the treadmill would go. Even if we just stood on the thing without moving, it would be a fun spot to look out our windows on pretty, snowy winter mornings.

I told Jeff what we had just ordered and said, "Who knows where it will lead?" Jeff, a purist in the purest sense of the word, is not a big fan of treadmills. He has run 25 marathons in his life and never once used a treadmill. But he is a runner and, like all runners, he encourages others as well to take up running—even if it happens to be on a treadmill. Then I mentioned that Anna and I had gotten married at the Bully Hill Winery on the same day they were running the Wineglass Marathon, and at the time I told Anna, "Someday I'll do that." She just said, "Yeah," and left it at that.

The Wineglass Marathon takes place in the middle of the Finger Lakes region, famous as New York State's wine country (hence the name of the marathon), and it is very pretty in the fall. Jeff knew this race well, as he had run it before on two different occasions. When I told him my story, he said that I should plan on giving it a shot. Others would have laughed, but he told me, "Just do it." *And why not?* I secretly thought. After all, our tenth wedding anniversary was coming up the following year. The timing couldn't have been better.

It was early November when the treadmill arrived. As this is bow-hunting season for me, it did not get much use at first. I did do a cursory walk on it to show Anna that we did not waste our money, but that was the extent of it. Still, while I was out hunting, I would spend my entire day in the tree stand thinking about running the marathon. The more I thought about it, the more I wanted to do it.

As soon as hunting season ended, I started using the treadmill. It was very awkward at first. I did not know what speed to start at. I kept sliding backwards, and would have slid off the back if not for the automatic turn-off, which activates when you fall. Even when I finally got the speed and rhythm down, I still did not know what incline to use. I was used to the elliptical machine, which I would set at two minutes low, then two minutes at just about the highest setting. But the settings for the treadmill did not work the same way, and it took me some time to figure it all out. Who would ever imagine that learning how to run could be so hard?

I made surprisingly good progress, and soon I was up to five miles a pop on the machine. It took me a whole hour to do that, which is certainly not a great pace—but at least I was running! But would I ever be ready for the real thing?

New Year's Eve was just around the corner, and Jeff and his wife were planning on celebrating the occasion in Saratoga Springs. He suggested that we run the First Night 5K race at Skidmore College. This is a very popular event, and it sounded like fun. And besides, it would give me an excuse to hang out with Jeff, so I agreed to accompany him.

Five kilometers equals three miles. I knew I could do that, because I was running five miles on the machine. Nevertheless, Jeff stressed that I really needed to run outdoors. He also told me to invest in a good pair of running shoes. I'm from the old school of footwear: one pair of Keds sneakers was sufficient for all my needs.* Jeff's advice was to visit the Fleet Feet store in Syracuse, New York. He said that they really knew their stuff and that, personally, he liked Brooks running shoes. Anna and I both agreed that maybe an official pair of running shoes would be better for my knees, so we headed off to Syracuse for the day to go shoe shopping.

Jeff was right: the salespeople at Fleet Feet really did know their stuff. First they measured my feet and watched me run on their little track. I tried on several different brands, eventually settling on a pair of Brooks, because they felt the most comfortable on my feet. The fact that a runner like Jeff liked them too was an extra reassurance on the wisdom of my choice. The only problem was that they cost $125. Never in my life have I spent that much money on a pair of shoes. Even the tango shoes I had custom-made for me in Argentina were less expensive. Here I am, a fully emancipated

---

* If I mention any specific shoe stores or brands from hereon in, please be aware that this does not represent any sort of product endorsement. It is important that athletes in the market for sneakers choose a pair that works for *them*.

57 year-old adult male—and I'm afraid my mother might be mad at me for wasting money on something so frivolous as a pair of sneakers. Sorry, mom! I took the plunge and brought them home. Thinner by $125, even my wallet was losing weight.

For some reason, however, I was extremely reluctant to take the Brooks out of the box. It was almost Christmas and I still had not run outside. In part, I didn't want to dirty up my expensive new shoes in the winter muck. More importantly, I felt very self-conscious about people watching me. After all, running is what young, thin, fit people do—not someone like me. Finally, on a cold, crisp day, I bit the bullet, drove to the nearby State Park, and mapped out a five-mile course for myself. Then I strapped on my old sneakers (the new running shoes were still safely ensconced inside their box) and started to run.

If nothing else, I learned something new that day: never run in the cold without gloves! I did my five miles and sweated a lot, but my fingers froze. I think this is one of the side effects of losing weight. No matter how warm my core is, now my fingers are always cold.

CƦՑꙨ

One of the things I do every year at Christmas time is bake cheesecake for my friends. I do make a pretty good cheesecake, if I do say so myself. One of the traditional recipients of this culinary largesse is my friend Jerry. We got to know each other years ago when we lived in the same housing development, watching our kids grow up together. Even though we don't see one another often, we have remained friends, and this is my way of staying in touch. When I delivered the cake to his house, he was stunned by how much weight I had lost. He hadn't seen me in months, and now I was down to 205 pounds. I mentioned to him that I planned on running the First Night race. He said that he had done it several years ago. Then he asked me, with worry in his voice, "You aren't going to try to do it in less than 30 minutes, right? I mean, that's *my* best time so far." I assured him that I would not, since it had taken me over an hour to run five miles.

New Years Eve finally arrived. The weather was particularly mild for this time of year (in upstate New York, it is not uncommon to have snow and bitterly cold temperatures on New Year's). This may sound funny, but had it been snowing, my new running shoes would have stayed in the box. As race time approached, I got dressed and put on my new shoes. The first thing I noticed when I stepped outside was that I could feel the cold air on my feet much more with these shoes. It turns they are made that way for ventilation to keep one's feet cool and dry while running. I hadn't thought about that before, so the mild weather was doubly fortuitous.

Anna drove me to the college and dropped me off at the staging area for the race. What a shock! The place was packed with people, and loud music was blaring from loudspeakers. There were young kids and old folks, dressed in every outfit imaginable. Some were stretching and warming up, while others were still putting on their number tags. Though the atmosphere was festive, I had a moment of panic. With 1,300 runners, how was I ever going to find Jeff? I looked all over and could not see him anywhere. Then, at the last minute (because things happen for a reason), Jeff's wife found me. I had met her only once before. How she recognized me, I will never know. She brought me over to where Jeff was waiting just before the race started. We took our place in crowd. He told me to pace myself, and to be careful not to burn out too fast. "Be a second-half runner," he said, using a term I would hear again and again from him. I was there just to have fun, but now I was starting to realize that people like Jeff really took this seriously.

The gun went off, and the crowd began to move. I did not appreciate it fully at the time, but this was an event that would change my life. I tried to have a conversation with Jeff, but he told me not to talk and to save my breath (something else I would hear again and again from him). All I knew was that I was running—and having fun, of course—but then something amazing happened. As we approached the one-mile mark, I noticed a big timing clock in front of me. The display read 11 minutes and a few seconds. I thought to myself, *Maybe, just maybe, I can beat Jerry.* At that moment I became competitive, and also began to take running seriously. I picked up speed. Jeff told me to hold back. He said we had a long way to go, and there were more hills ahead. I listened to him out of respect for his experience; but inside, I wanted to explode and let loose.

At the two-mile mark, the clock said 20 minutes. *I could do this.* I wanted it so bad that I picked up my pace, and this time Jeff did not hold back either. We rounded the corner together and headed up the last street. One more mile. But here was the hill Jeff had warned me about. We pushed on and reached the top. I was gasping for air. Now I knew why you don't talk during a race. We made a left turn onto the college campus. The music was growing louder, and the cheers of the crowd were louder still. In the distance I could see the finish line. The clock said 29 something, but it was a blur. I kept running, faster, faster. In the last 25 yards, I watched Jeff pull in front of me. I was glad to see this, because I knew he would have had a much faster race, but he had held back to be with me, his friend the novice runner. He deserved to win. Nevertheless, I dug down deep for my last reserves of strength, and in a final burst of speed I crossed the finish line at 29 minutes 29 seconds. I had done it. I had completed my first race. *And I had beaten Jerry!* More importantly, I was hooked for life. I was now a runner.

After I crossed the finish line, someone hung a ribbon with a medal on it around my neck. It was an unremarkable-looking token of a relatively modest achievement; but to me, it felt like Olympic gold. I took the medal home, showed it off proudly to Anna, and hung it over the fireplace, where it remains to this day among all the others I have collected since then. But this was my first, and so it takes pride of place on the wall. I also saved the racing bib—that piece of waterproof fabric with a runner's number printed on it, which you pin onto your shirt or shorts when you race. It has a special chip built into it that records your time. I save each one from my races and write the date and my time on the back of them. I am happy to say that I have since accumulated a nice little collection of these bibs. This one, however—First Night 2011—is the one that lies at the top of the pile.

So now that I was hooked on running, what next? Jeff told me to do more 5K races and to think about the Wineglass Marathon in October. Was I really ready to commit to that? Maybe not quite yet. But not a second went by that I did not think about it.

CRSO

The winter of 2011 was long, cold, and snowy. I gave the treadmill quite a workout that season. I knew that if I harbored any hope of running a marathon, I would need to increase both my distance and my endurance. So I pushed myself harder each day. My visits to the Y became less frequent, because I spent all my time on the treadmill. By the middle of February I was running 8 miles in just less than two hours. I knew that my speed would be a problem, but I had always been a slow runner. That is what had dissuaded me from ever considering a marathon before. If I let that get in the way now, I would be sunk. Instead, I focused on the positive. For one thing, I could run for eight miles, which in and of itself is no mean feat. My weight, now close to 200, continued to drop too. No matter where I was, no matter what I was doing, if I was not concentrating on a task, my thoughts would wander to the previously unthinkable: *Is it possible? Can I really run a marathon?*

I began searching the Internet for information on marathons. I found training logs and nutritional advice, personal blogs and advertisements galore for products aimed at runners. There was something for everybody, and too much for any one person. I felt like a kid in a candy shop. I could not consume enough of these runners' "goodies." One day I looked up the Boston Marathon. I had always thought of that event as the gold standard of marathons. It is by far the most famous that I knew about. Hell, they even cover it live on TV, so it must a big deal. Don't get me wrong: I had no illusions about running the Boston Marathon. I just thought it would be a good place to begin my research on the topic.

I knew about the Wineglass too, of course, but wanted to see what else there was. It did not take long before I found several web-sites with a list of all the marathons in the country and their dates. As I scrolled down the list, starting in January, I noticed that none of them were held nearby. All the winter marathons took place in states to the south and west. The closer I got to April on the calendar, however, the more they began to crop up in New York and the northeast. By June there were very few listed anywhere, right through the summer; by the fall, though, I saw more and more of them on the list, moving from north to south. This was a revelation to me. Yet, if you stop to think about it, this makes perfect sense. In the summer, it is too hot to run that far, so most marathons tend to be scheduled for the cooler times of the year.

I had already confided in Jeff that I was seriously contemplating running the Wineglass, but I did not tell anyone else. How would I manage it? I was not even remotely sure that it was possible for me. But the thought of it gave some solidity to my dreams. Then one day, while looking over the list of upcoming races, I noticed two listed in Vermont. One took place in Burlington, while the other was run from Bennington to

Manchester. Both were scheduled for the middle of May. The latter one was called the Shires of Vermont Marathon, and this was the very first year they were running it. A "shire," by the way, is any meadowland between hills. When Vermont was first settled, it was divided into the North Shire and the South Shire. Bennington lay in the south and Manchester in the north. Hence the name, "The Shires of Vermont."

Southern Vermont and east-central New York (along the Vermont border) are Anna's and my favorite part of the country. Cows fill the open meadows surrounded by rolling hills, and maple syrup shacks dot the landscape. There are cheese shops and antique shops and art studios and—well, I can go on and on. It is like something out of a Norman Rockwell painting. In fact, until recently the Norman Rockwell Museum was located in Arlington, Vermont, before it moved to its permanent home over the border in Stockbridge, Massachusetts. The famous New England folk art painter Grandma Moses has a museum in her birth town of Bennington.

The famed Battenkill River, one of the most storied fly-fishing rivers in the east, starts in the mountains outside Manchester. It starts as a freestone stream and flows past the Orvis flagship store and fly rod shop in Manchester. To those who know nothing of such things, this may not seem important. But to those of us who like to fish, this is hallowed ground. The Battenkill is also my favorite trout stream anywhere. The fishing is nowhere near as spectacular as it once was, when three- and four-pounders were common, and a fish over five pounds was not unheard of. Nowadays, thanks to acid rain and a whole host of other issues, the quality of the fishing has greatly declined over the past decades. Things are slowly changing for the better, however. On the Vermont side of the river, no fish have been stocked for years. Any fish you catch are wild brown trout born and bred in the river. They are colorful, strong, and feisty. To catch one, particularly on a dry fly, is a wonderful experience. The first few miles of river on the New York side are designated catch-and-release only. It is stocked every year with a healthy number of large brown trout, which results in some great fishing.

The race was scheduled for May 17—exactly 1 year and 2 days since the day I had gone to see the nutritionist for the first time. That kudu hiding in the brush was getting restless. I started to think, *My God, is this possible?* I quickly dismissed such thoughts as little more than a pipedream, a matter of too much, too soon. I had not even run my second 5K race, yet here I was seriously contemplating a marathon. Try as I might to push the thought to the back of my mind, it refused to go quietly. I often found myself imagining what it would be like to run through that beautiful countryside, to run through those quaint towns, to run though all that colonial history.

I decided that I would tell Jeff about this marathon and see what he thought about it. In hopes of encouraging him to agree that it was a good idea, I put the most positive spin possible on my description of the event, pointing out that I would be running through some of the most idyllic countryside around and right alongside the scenic Battenkill River, with its native brown trout cheering me on.

Jeff wouldn't buy any of it. "Hold your horses! You're not ready yet for such a long run." He encouraged me instead to focus on the Wineglass in the fall. He insisted—and rightly so—that a person should train for six months to a year for a marathon; and reiterated that I should do more short races first, working my way up from 5Ks to 15Ks. He assured me that I was doing well with my training but needed additional time and training before I tackled more ambitious runs. He was correct on every count. I hung up the phone, feeling a little dejected, but trusting his judgment. He is a fool who does not heed a wise man's advice.

Days came and went, and I made the best of my disappointment. Yet with every mile I ran on the treadmill, all that I could picture in my mind's eye was the Vermont countryside rolling by. For months I had been consumed with running a marathon, any marathon; now I was consumed with running this one in particular, the Shires. Try as I might, I could not get it out of my mind. What a quandary. On the one hand, I knew I should listen to my experienced friend. On the other, I do much better when I have short-term goals in front of me. The Wineglass in October was too far away for me to focus on. What should I do?

Once again, the invisible hand of fate helped me decide.

㈲

The company my wife works for has several offices in the United States and around world. There is an office in Saratoga Springs, another in Chicago, as well as a software development center in India and a data entry center in Montego Bay, Jamaica. Anna is in charge of the people in India and supervises several people in Jamaica. They recently hired a few more people in the Jamaica office and needed to get them trained quickly. We were both pleasantly surprised to learn that the company wanted to send her there for a week at the end of February, putting her up in an all-inclusive resort on the beach. She would still have to put in 40 hours training the new people; but at least there were plenty of amenities to enjoy in between times. As "working vacations" go, this was not a bad deal—especially for me! Except for the price of a mere plane ticket, I could come along and enjoy those amenities for free.

With snow—measured in feet—piling up outside and the temperatures well below freezing, this unexpected mid-winter getaway came as a welcome relief. I had not run outside since New Year's Eve and looked forward to trading in the stationary monotony of a treadmill for the sight of passing palm trees waving under sunny, blue skies. Just before we left, I gave Jeff another call to see if he had reconsidered his original advice. He had not. He remained adamant in his opinion that I wait until the fall before trying a marathon. This time, however, he added that if I really wanted to give it a whirl, he would not stand in my way. I was still at sixes and sevens about it. Yet my friend, while he still did not fully sanction my desire, at least offered me some kind of loophole.

The morning of our trip arrived—and along with it, yet more snow and slippery roads. I should have been thinking about Jamaica; but during the tense, quiet drive to Albany International, all I could picture in my mind was Vermont. Never mind the flight departing on time, or even at all; we would be lucky just to make it to the airport. As it happens, we *were* lucky: the snow turned to rain in Albany, and our plane took off without delay. The first half of the flight was bumpy as we flew over the storm, but then it settled down. We changed planes in Charlotte and were soon Jamaican-bound.

As you may have guessed, I am an impatient fellow, and so I looked for ways to make the time pass more quickly. Plucking the in-flight magazine from the seat pocket in front of me, I began absentmindedly leafing through it. On one of the pages I noticed a picture of Mark Twain accompanied by one of the famous quotes frequently (but incorrectly) ascribed to him: "Twenty years from now you will be more disappointed by the things that you didn't do than by the ones you did do. So throw off the bowlines. Sail away from the safe harbor. Catch the trade winds in your sails. Explore. Dream. Discover." Even if he didn't actually say this, it's a good quote, and I could not get it out of my head.

On the taxi ride from Sangster International Airport to the resort, I took mental snapshots of the places we passed in and around Montego Bay, so that later I could map out a good running route. If you like sun, sand, and palm trees (oh, and rum, of course), Jamaica is *the* place to be. I felt bad that my wife would miss out on some of the fun, as she had to work during the day; but I fully intended to make the most of my time here.

The next morning, as soon as Anna left for the office, I changed into my running clothes and headed toward the main entrance of the resort. Before I even started to run, a tall, lanky Jamaican man stepped out of a car parked just outside the front gate and asked how far I was going to run. I did not feel unsafe, but certainly thought it odd. Then he asked if I wanted something to help me run, whereupon he pulled out a handful of joints. I could not help but smile. He was the local ganja dealer, just plying his trade. You'll find one in front of every hotel here. After all, pot is legal in Jamaica. I almost bought one of his wares, just to support the local economy; but since cannabis is not part of my training plan, I passed on it.

I started down the road. The warmth and sunshine were a far cry from the weather in upstate New York. Best of all, I was running *outside* again. Life was good—even without the help of pot. My goal was to run to the center of town and back. The day before, as our driver took us through Montego Bay, I had noticed a KFC restaurant on one of the street corners. It was hard to miss the giant bucket above the red building. I remembered how fried chicken used to be one of my favorite foods. That was a different time, though, and now my life revolved around eating right and exercising. Still, it was a good landmark to aim for.

The streets of Jamaica are narrow, and the sidewalks even narrower. People also drive on the left side of the road. Jamaican drivers are plainly crazy, and I firmly believe they take great pride in trying to hit as many tourists as they can. As least they do you the courtesy of beeping before they run you down. I learned very quickly to move out of the way whenever I heard a horn blow behind me.

I made it to the KFC without incident—about 2½ miles I figured—and started the return leg of my run. I was about a half mile from the hotel when I came upon another runner. I was closing the distance on him and thought I might be able to pass him. I was feeling proud of myself, maybe even a little cocky, and considered turning around and running the route again. God has a way of keeping you humble, though. Mind you, I was not going very fast or pushing myself terribly hard; but all of a sudden I felt a disturbing tightness in the back of my left leg. At first I thought I could just run it out. After a few yards more, however, the tightness turned to spasms of pain, as if someone had kicked me in the muscle midway between the hip and knee. I slowed to a walk and watched the runner in front of me pull away. The pain went away. But as soon as I started to run again, it came back. What was going on? I repeated this scenario about three times before I gave up and limped past the pot dealer into the resort.

After a quick shower, I got on the Internet and googled "pain in the back of your leg." After a few minutes of research, it became clear that I had pulled a hamstring—which isn't exactly helpful. That vague description covers most types of pain one can experience in the muscles of the thigh's posterior. One article noted that if the hamstring is torn, there will be a large bruise visible on the surface that may take months to heal. I did not notice any black and blue marks on my leg, so I figured that it was only slightly strained and would surely be better by the next day.

Tomorrow came, and my leg felt fine. Nevertheless, I thought it the better part of valor to give it a rest. After Anna left for work, I decided to skip running, and instead went to the health club and got on the elliptical machine. I started out slow, and was prepared to stop at the first sign of pain. There was none. I pushed a little harder. Still none. Now I went faster and increased the resistance. Nothing. Whatever the problem was, seemingly it had passed.

The next morning, I was ready to try again. I headed out the front gate and was greeted by the pot dealer. He asked, "How far today?" and, optimist that I am, I answered, "Ten miles." I reached the end of the road. So far, so good. Then I turned left toward the center of town, and about 100 yards down the road the pain began again. It hurt too much to continue running. I walked under a tree and tried stretching. The pain stopped. As soon as I tried running again, however, it came back with a vengeance. I thought to myself, *Screw this, I'm going to run through it.*

Now, let me give you a bit of advice. If you are experiencing any severe physical pain, it means your body is trying to tell you that something is wrong. Pushing yourself is not going to help, and very likely it will exacerbate the problem. As I began to run again, I suddenly felt something snap. I froze, not from the pain but rather from the fear that I had done some real damage to myself. Less than fifteen minutes after I had told him I intended to run ten miles, I limped past the pot dealer, a hangdog expression on my face. Back in my room I carefully looked the leg over. There was no sign of bruising, but I knew I wouldn't be running anymore on this trip.

For now I would have to stick to the elliptical machine in the health club. I decided to really push myself on it and build up my endurance. Instead of a one-hour workout, I would try two. The next morning I showed up at the health club right at 6:00, when they opened up. I knew it would not be busy for a while and that no one would mind if I monopolized the Cybex machine. I put in my ear buds, queued up some tunes, and started exercising.

The health club occupied a big, open space filled with the usual things one would find in a fitness center. The walls had tinted glass to keep out the hot rays of the sun, and the side windows offered a view of the recreational area beside the pool. From where I stood I could see thatched umbrellas surrounding the pool. In the middle of the pool was a bar you could swim out to, and stools in the water to sit on while you drank. In the afternoon, a DJ played reggae music while bikini-clad college girls danced on the patio. Now the place was quiet. Beyond the pool, a palm-shaded beach dropped off gently to meet the warm, green Caribbean. Just a few days ago I had been up to my knees in snow, and now I was in paradise. Despite the slight setback with my leg, truly I felt like a blessed man at that moment.

The first hour of the workout went well. I could detect no hint of the pain that had sidelined me from running. Which struck me as odd. The two exercises—running outside and running on the elliptical machine—use the same muscles and involve virtually identical movements. Yet one caused pain and one did not. After an hour, I stopped and drank some water, refilled my bottle, and changed my sweatband. I did not know how long I could go for, but if I did not have the endurance to last two hours here, how on earth could I hope to run 26 miles? I climbed back onto the machine and programmed in another hour-long workout.

The second hour went even better. By the time the timer counted away the last few seconds, I felt sweaty and hot, but my muscles knew they had accomplished something. They tingled all over, but it was a good sensation, one of strength rather than exhaustion. This was what I was hoping for. For the rest of the day my mood could only be described as jubilant. It is amazing what a couple hours of endorphins will do for you.

The next day I decided to really push myself and try for a three-hour workout. At a minimum, that level of endurance is what a marathon requires. I did not want to tie up the machine for three hours straight during the morning, when everyone else would be using the equipment, so I planned on starting at 11:00 A.M. Breakfast was long over, and lunchtime was at least an hour away. When I arrived, I had the place all to myself.

The first hour ticked by, a carbon copy of the previous day's workout. By the time the second hour got underway, I realized my zeal for the enterprise was beginning to wane. How long can a person stand in one place, putting one foot in front of the other over and over again, but without getting anywhere? No matter how pretty the view, such repetition becomes boring after a while. To stay focused and alert, I would have to ignore the scenery and look inward, concentrating on my rhythm and my timing and my speed. It may seem like a little thing, but it was this kind of mental discipline, not feats of strength, that would lay the foundation of workouts to come.

I was glad when the second hour ended. How could I possibly do another? Two days of hard exercise had drained my reserves of energy. But I wanted this. I needed this. So I refilled the water bottle, changed my sweatband again, grabbed a dry towel, and programmed one more hour into the machine. Now we would see what I was *really* made of.

What I discovered at the end of that third hour is that I was made of sweat and muscle, determination and grit—all the qualities required of a marathon runner. My legs felt wobbly as I stepped off the machine. I had never before worked so hard for so long. I had become severely overheated and hypoglycemic. I drank deep and often, refilling the water bottle only to empty it again immediately. If had known then what I know now about carbo-loading and glycogen stores and energy gel packs, the day would have turned out much different. But I didn't. It took my last ounce of strength to walk out to the pool and fall in, clothes and all.

Before we returned to the snow-bound north, I did several more two-hour workouts and one three-hour workout. I had been able to spend that much time exercising only because I was on vacation and thus enjoyed the luxury of plenty of free time. I had proven to myself that I had a good enough physical foundation to build on, not to mention a commitment to succeed. But the commitment of time was another story. With my work schedule, how would I manage to do the same back home? That question nagged at me now—along with the fact that apparently I could not run 50 yards unless I was on an elliptical machine. For good or ill, marathons take place on solid ground, not on machines.

As we boarded the plane to return home, my mind was filled with all that had happened during the last week. We taxied down the runway and lifted off, circling over the green water with its whitecap waves and dark coral reefs, and headed north. Somewhere over Cuba I started leafing through the airline's in-flight magazine again, until I came to the page with Mark Twain's picture and that quote staring me in the face. Twenty years from now, did I want to feel disappointment over the things I had not done—or triumph for having done them? I knew the odds were stacked against me. True, it would be physically hard and would demand a very large commitment of my time. But could I do it? Could I really run a marathon? I already knew the answer to that question. Yes, I could. I wanted to do it. At the very least, I wanted to try. I wanted it so bad, I could taste it. Odds be damned: I decided then and there to give it my best shot.

As with most decisions, I felt better after I had made this one. The mental debate was over and now I could focus on the future. It may have been summer-like in Jamaica, but here in upstate New York it was still decidedly winter; and so my immediate future involved shoveling lots of snow once we got home. We quickly settled back into our respective routines, with Anna working from home, while I would travel to Syracuse to work for three days and return home for four. My first morning back from Syracuse, I woke up early and headed for the Y, where I did two hours on the elliptical. The next day I ran two hours on the treadmill next to

Anna's desk. I took a break from exercising on Sunday, but Monday I was back at the Y. This time I did three hours on the elliptical. When I returned home, Anna got curious. "Why were you gone so long?"

I had not yet told her about my decision. She had no idea I was even thinking about running a marathon, much less that I had already signed up for the Shires of Vermont. I had even started a training log to mark my progress.

The next week played out the same way; and upon returning from the Y, I was met with the same inquisitive look from Anna. You can imagine what might have been going through her mind. Her hubby has lost considerable weight, and now he uncharacteristically disappears for hours at a time. I don't think she really suspected me of anything dishonorable, but one could hardly blame her if she did.

I knew I would have to tell her my plans eventually, but was at first reluctant to do so because of the expected response. "You'll get hurt. It's too much. It's too far. And what about your heart?" These were all valid points, and she would have been right on all of them. I just didn't want to hear them, so I kept her in the dark. But I knew I had to tell her sometime. It was the middle of March, and in a few days she would be traveling back to Russia to visit her father. How could I let her go abroad, not knowing what I was up to? Now was as good a time as any to tell her.

It was a sunny Saturday afternoon. I was sitting outside on our porch, studying the race website, when Anna came out to join me. I closed the computer and asked her to sit down. I had something to tell her. "You know all the training I've been doing? Well, here's why." And then I told her about my plans.

Her response was just what I had expected. "It's too far." "It's too much." "How about shorter races first?" On and on she went. I listened to her objections, and then explained my thoughts. We played verbal ping-pong for a while, until finally I promised not to do anything stupid. At the first sign of injury, or worse, I would stop. She seemed satisfied with this compromise—most likely because she figured that the chances of my running a marathon were so remote, it was a waste of her time to argue about it. We agreed that I could continue exercising, she would monitor my progress, and we would discuss it again later.

"Later" came the next morning. It was Sunday, and we had planned on taking our annual pilgrimage to have breakfast at a maple syrup shack on the Vermont border. I got up early and hit the treadmill right away—mainly to burn off some calories before feasting on pancakes. By now I was running pretty well: in just over two hours I could do 12 miles. When I told Anna that I had just run almost half a marathon, something changed. I could see it in her eyes. She was thinking, *This is possible. He just might be able to do it.* After that, she never used the words "Too far" again.

On March 23, Anna left to visit her father. The next day my marathon training, already underway, began in earnest.

CHAPTER 3

Marathon Training Log

DAY 1

March 11 — Saratoga Springs

I have not worked out since leaving Jamaica four days ago. Today I went to the Y and did three hours on the Advantage machine. I was only planning on doing two; but I felt good, so I did the extra. I most likely could have done a fourth hour, but I needed more water and did not want to overdo it.

The hamstring is not too bad; however, when I move just the right way, I can feel it tightening up. I started doing stretches today and will try to do that several times a day. That may help.

I also signed up for the Shires of Vermont Marathon today. It takes place on May 15, beginning in Bennington, Vermont, continuing through Arlington, then along the Battenkill River to Manchester. That area is one of my favorite places. It is also close to the one-year anniversary, almost to the day, of my improved diet and new lifestyle. It seems fitting that I aim for this goal. The only problem is that right now I still can't run more than 100 yards because of my hamstring. But I *know* I can do this.

DAY 2
March 12 — Saratoga Springs

Swam 1 hour today.

DAY 3
March 13 — Saratoga Springs

Did two hours on the Cybex machine. This is the same type of machine the resort had at the health club in Jamaica. I like this machine, although the handles are different on this one. My arms do not swing so far, and it does not read your pulse. But I feel it gives me a much better workout than the Advantage machine. Or at any rate I sweat more.

Hamstring still feels tight, but I'm stretching it often.

DAY 4

March 14 — Saratoga Springs

Went to the Y today. Had big plans, but things didn't go the way I had hoped. I wanted to do a few hours on the Cybex, but just lacked the energy to follow through. I was getting a friction rub too, so I stopped after an hour.

DAY 5

March 16 — Syracuse

Woke up in the apartment at 4:30 today. Got up and had coffee and yogurt first. Read my email and then did one hour on the NordicTrack. This machine is a godsend. I could feel it stretch my hamstring, and now I'm hooked on it. It made my leg feel much better. I'm almost tempted to bring it back home with me to Saratoga. I still stretch a few times during the day, and the leg is steadily improving. I'm actually thinking about running again without the machine. It is hard to hold off, but I will give the leg one more week's respite.

DAY 6
March 17 — Syracuse

Happy St. Patrick's Day! Had to pack up and leave early today, so I did only 30 minutes on the NordicTrack. It felt good to move, but I had to stop just as I was getting warmed up. I gave both legs a good stretching. The right one feels tighter than the left, but there is no pain to speak of. Maybe the hamstring really is healing.

DAY 7
March 18 — Saratoga

Woke up early today and stretched before going to the Y. I have come to the conclusion that this is as important as putting on my running shoes. I will never exercise again without stretching first.

I discovered a newer version of the Cybex machine at the Y— a superior model in most respects. What I liked best about it is that it has a built-in fan. Every exercise machine should have one. What I did not like is that I could not set the upper resistance to 50 exactly. It kept defaulting to 55, which was too much for me, and I had to stop and lower it every time the resistance increased. It also forces me to do 1 minute up and 1 minute down. The older ones do 30 seconds up and 1½ minutes down. No more slacking off, I guess!

I did three hours on this new Cybex. Feeling tight during the first hour, I fought the urge to abandon it for the rest of the day. The second hour went quicker, so I did a third hour. For the last 10 or 15 minutes, I really turned on the speed.

I'm pretty convinced that I could have done a fourth hour. If I had had something to eat, I probably would have. I need to eat more before the workout, or maybe after the third hour. Although I sweated up a storm, it did not seem excessive. The fan helped a lot. I don't know how this exercise compares to actual running; but if it is even remotely similar, I think I just might be able to run the full 26 miles.

A funny thing happened when I first arrived at the Y today. Inside the locker that I picked to stow my clothes in today, I discovered a packet of energy gel. This is a high-calorie, electrolyte-rich goo designed to give athletes a quick energy boost during an intense workout. I had no idea such things existed. Did someone leave it behind by accident—or was it a secret gift from my kudu?

DAY 8

March 19 — Saratoga

I tried something new. Instead of exercising first thing in the morning, I did it in the afternoon. It is hard for me to stop what I'm doing in the middle of the day; but when I exercise then, I feel more relaxed, more limber, and better fed. The latter has become more important to me, because I can't exercise without fuel. So at around 2:00 P.M. I got all dressed up in my new running attire, new running underwear, and my usual bandanna, and wore both knee braces this time. I felt a little like a Samurai warrior.

Prepared for battle now, I stepped onto the treadmill and started off at a walking pace of 4 miles/hour and increased it from there. I was very worried that my leg might start hurting. Every time I felt the slightest twinge, my guts churned and I thought, *Here it comes*. But the pain didn't come, so I gradually increased the speed in half-mile increments, from 4½ miles to 6 miles/hour. At that speed, technically, I wasn't walking on the treadmill, but *running*. Whenever I started to feel my left hamstring tightening up, I decreased the speed, and the pain went away. Then I would ratchet up the speed again until the next twinge. Sometimes I had to slow myself down to a brisk walk, as I did not want push my luck and re-injure myself.

I had the machine set for a 500-calorie goal. It took about 48 minutes to reach it. By the time I did, my thigh was feeling better. After a short break, I got on the treadmill again. Anna thought I should have stopped here so as not to hurt my leg, but I wanted to see what would happen. Nothing did, so I started on my second 500-calorie workout on the machine.

After about 15 minutes, I could feel the hamstring start to loosen up. I ran slowly, between 5 and 5½ miles/hour. The hamstring kept threatening to hurt, but by favoring that leg I got though the workout without pain. The effort, however, had left me exhausted. I needed fluids, a new shirt, and some calories. I swigged down some Gatorade, followed by a protein shake. The nourishment helped revive me, so I decided to work off another 500 calories.

At the end of three hours, I felt tired. I noticed that with each workout, it was taking less and less time for me to reach my goal. Burning off the last 500 calories took only 45 minutes. Moreover, my distance increased from 4.1 to 4.25 miles/500 calories. In other words, I had run the equivalent of 12½ miles—which is almost half the length of a marathon!

DAY 9
March 24 — Saratoga

When I drove back from Syracuse last night, I measured a stretch of road near my house that I wanted to run. It loops from Route 29 to Kirby Road and home from there—a seven-mile round trip exactly. Perfect. My plan is to do the 7 miles once, just to see how I make out. Then I will work my way up to 14 miles and eventually to 21 miles, with a break in between to drink something and change my shirt.

After a good night's rest, I dressed in my winter running clothes and did the 7 miles in about 70 minutes. I felt great afterward and was reasonably happy with my time.

DAY 10
March 26 — Saratoga

Paid a visit to my nutritionist after my last run. She gave me a plan to follow so I can take in enough calories to keep up my endurance. She advised me to eat before I run, to stop frequently, and to drink plenty of fluids. She recommended the running gels, and also suggested that I carbo-load on the morning of my runs.

Today I woke up, drank my coffee, stretched, and (following the nutritionist's advice) ate a cup of oatmeal. That filled me up.

Now I was ready. I got dressed, set my timer, and began to run. Every now and then I felt a twinge in my hamstring, but it passed quickly. Not wanting to push it, I kept my speed at about 6 miles/hour, and made it back home in 86 minutes. Not as good a time as I had hoped, but good enough. I planned on doing a second lap, and maybe even a third.

Drank a liter of Gatorade, changed my shirt, reset the timer, and set out again. It is hard to get started after resting. I was hobbling like an old man. Once I warmed up, though, my stride smoothed out. I was halfway down Grand Avenue when I began to get a little tired. Once I reached the hill at the very end of the road, my body was running on empty. I kept repeating to myself, "This is bad, but you can do it." And after a time, I did do it. A profound sense of pride filled my being. Cresting the top of the hill, I felt like Rocky jumping up and down at the top of the Philadelphia Museum steps, holding his arms up in triumph.

Now to head back home. By the time I reached the bottom of the hill, I could no longer feel my legs. They weren't numb, exactly. They just felt like they were not there, as if the wind was blowing through where my legs should be, while the rest of my body floated on a cushion of air.

I still planned on doing the third lap. But the more I ran, the more tired I got. Besides, by now my right big toe was beginning to hurt. When I got home and pulled off my sock, I saw that the nail had somehow gotten pushed up and back. I decided I was done for the day. I had run 14 miles (which is more than half a marathon), and I was happy with that. I just wish I could have done it faster, or had a little more strength in reserve at the end.

DAY 11
March 27 — Saratoga

Woke up with big plans, but reality intervened. To begin with, my big toe was still sore and had turned black and blue under the nail. It looked worse than it felt. I trimmed the nail and put on a few Band-Aids. Did my morning routine and then started running. My throat burned, and my lungs coughed up phlegm. *This is strange*, I thought. *Maybe I'm getting sick.* I could only manage one seven-mile lap. After yesterday's triumph, I returned home feeling a little dejected, licking my wounds. I consoled myself with the knowledge that at least I had run the seven miles, which is better than nothing. Now I realize that after a long 14-mile run like yesterday's, I should have rested a day.

After this I got progressively sicker.

DAY 12
April 1 — Saratoga

Despite feeling ill, I worked 48 hours over four days in
Syracuse, then stayed a fifth day and worked six hours more. I
packed up and got home around 5:00 P.M. and was on the treadmill
by 6:00. The first three miles were rough, and I coughed up green
phlegm the whole way. After that I started to come around, though;
and by the end of my eighth mile, I felt pretty good. I only stopped
because of the time. It was now 7:30, and I had not eaten yet. I was
happy with the distance but not the speed. I'm beginning to think I
may never run faster than 5½ miles/hour.

DAY 13
April 2 — Saratoga

Too cold and wet to run outside. I ate, stretched, and started to
run on the treadmill. The first three miles went better than
yesterday, but not great. I'm still coughing up crap. After the first
seven miles, I had a faint surge of optimism. I did stop at the five-
mile mark and drank some Gatorade, then started up again. I was
slowly getting into a comfortable groove.

After the next four miles, I slowed to a walk for a few minutes
and then started running again. I ran one more mile, stopped, and

drank. Maybe I was stopping too often or drinking too much; for whatever reason, I had a hard time getting back into the groove. My belly felt like it had a bowling ball sitting in it. I reached the 12-mile mark (1,500 calories), but just could not go on.

Feeling kind of discouraged now, I realized that I run too slow and make too many stops to finish within the six hours allotted for the race. Much as I would like to believe otherwise, perhaps sheer desire and determination alone are not enough to get me through 26 miles. For the first time since I started pursuing this dream, real doubt is setting in.

Doubt is a poison that seeps slowly into your veins and pollutes your thoughts. It is an assassin that stalks you in the dark, until suddenly it leaps up from its hiding place and stares you in the face, a malevolent enemy ready to strike you down. I don't know what will happen. I will keep trying, but let's face facts. I am 57 years old, and my body is well past its prime. If I keep doing this, it is only because I am too stupid to know when to throw in the towel.

DAY 14
April 7 — Saratoga

Thirty-seven days to go until the Big Race. I rested all week from running, and now this old carcass of mine is grateful for the respite. My right ankle had really been bothering me, so I paid a visit to the Fleet Feet store, and they fixed me up. When I told the sales associate that I had a case of posterior tibial tendonitis, he showed me a kit that would take care of that. The kit comes with a six-inch-high rubber block and another piece that looks something like a small dumbbell. You're supposed to put the dumbbell on the block and then roll your ankle over it using different ranges of motion. The kit, which costs $70, is designed to break up any adhesions. Skeptic that I am, I thought it was bogus; but what did I have to lose (besides $70)? I needed something, so I bought it. Will wonders never cease? The damn thing worked! By the next morning, the ankle felt 50% better, and the next day the problem was practically all cleared up. It still hurts a tiny bit, but is definitely much improved.

Today I decided to run in Saratoga National Historical Park, where the Revolutionary Army won a crucial victory over the British forces in 1777. The park has a tour road that is in good shape—unlike Grand Ave., where the pavement is broken and pitted. With one-way traffic in a single lane, next to a separate bike lane, drivers can't go above 20 mph, so it's fairly safe for runners.

I prepared two liters of Gatorade and another two liters of water, packed half a dozen energy gels, and brought along a tuna salad for lunch. Before heading out, I made sure to eat a good carbo-loading breakfast. My plan was to trace the route by car and leave a few water bottles for myself at strategic spots along the route. Unfortunately, today the road was closed to automobile traffic for some reason, so that brilliant idea had to be shelved. On to Plan B: keep my provisions in the car, and eat and drink in between laps.

I have a new app on my iPhone called *MapMyRun*, which is supposed to keep track of my exact distance and time. This would be my lengthiest run under "real world" conditions, if everything went as planned. The road is nine miles long, with a side loop of another mile. I hoped to run it twice, for a total of 20 miles. Toward the end of the route is a mile-long hill. My idea was to run the course in reverse. That way, I would start by going downhill rather than finishing it with an uphill slog. I really wanted to finish the full 20 miles, so I had no problem stacking the deck a little in my favor.

The plan looked good on paper. Once I reached the bottom of the hill, however, I realized that the course would not be as easy as expected. I seem to have forgotten that what goes up must come down—and vice versa. After that first gravity-assisted mile, I encountered a series of uphill climbs the entire rest of the way. They proved to be no serious obstacle, I am happy to report. At about the six-mile mark, a mile-long loop brought me to a very pretty overlook on the Hudson River, where the American forces had placed their cannons. Here it is all downhill one way and uphill the other, followed by another big hill. This leg of the run was a challenge, but I did fine. Two more miles and I would be back where I started. By now, the sweat was pouring off me like water from a spigot.

Ten miles down, ten to go! Back at the car, I didn't bother to eat anything, because I had taken a gel pack before the big hill and was not feeling hypoglycemic. I did drink a liter of Gatorade, though—and not a drop more. When I drank too much the last time, I had felt too bloated to run, so I was careful to limit my fluid intake before I began the second lap.

The first lap had taken a lot out of me—but far from everything. I felt enthusiastic if not optimistic, and so took it easy on the way down the first hill. It is 1¾ miles to the turn-off before the course starts its first uphill climb. At around the 12-mile mark the road levels off for a while, and I was still doing okay. It is hard to count the markers when going against the normal flow, but it was around mile 14 that I slowed to a walk. I probably could have kept up my speed, but I wanted to save something for the end.

Several times I alternated between walking and running. It felt better to run, because the more I ran, the quicker I would be done; so I ran as much as I could. I can't really say that my muscles hurt at all, but the tendons in my groin area were tightening up and starting to feel sore. But it was a good soreness, the kind you get when you've given yourself a solid workout.

It was somewhere around mile 15 that I realized just how dehydrated I had become. This was one of the spots where I had planned on leaving a water bottle for myself (if the road hadn't been closed to traffic). That water sure would have come in handy now! I had more energy gels, but my mouth was so dry that I didn't feel like eating them. Besides, thirst was the problem, not lack of fuel.

Now I had to make a decision: do I take the loop and run almost another mile before I hit the big hill, or do I skip the loop altogether and just call it a day? I had set 20 miles as my goal, and I was determined to stick to it. I turned left toward the loop, and that is when I started to fade fast. Worse yet, the sartorius muscle in my right leg—the longest one in the human body, which runs down the length of the thigh—began to go into spasms. I would walk it off for a minute and then start running again. Finally, even walking did no good. I stood there watching this one muscle quiver uncontrollably.

I could not stop it. All I could do was stare in disbelief. The entire muscle felt like one big charley horse.

After a brief rest, the muscle settled down, and I was able to walk the last two miles back to the car. At least I had covered the full 20 miles. But I really think that if had had more water to drink, my performance would have been much better.

DAY 15
April 9 — Saratoga

Planned a ten-mile run in Saratoga. Got up early, drove the route, and dropped off some bottles of water and Gatorade at various spots. Back at home I dressed, stretched, and started running. It felt good.

At the end of the first mile I passed by my old house. At 1.5 miles I passed the Y. I reached the first water bottle at 3 miles, but I didn't feel like drinking. The water was too cold, and I was not dehydrated yet. The next mile and a half was along a rough back road. Usually there's not too much traffic here, but it was change-of-shift time at the industrial park nearby, so I had to watch for oncoming cars.

I turned left at Grand Ave. I had left a water bottle for myself at the end of this stretch. I drank half the bottle, finished the last hill (which seemed steeper than I remembered), and drank the other half at the bottom. Three more miles, and I'm home.

Though I was working hard, I was far from exhausted. I kept up a steady pace and even tried to speed up at times. Once at home, I felt fine. Not too tired, not too thirsty. If I can work my way up to feeling this good doing 18 miles, I will surely be ready for 26.

Day 16
April 12 — Saratoga

Tried running the Battlefield route again. The tour road would be open this time, so I could leave my water bottles along the way. The road didn't open until 9:00 A.M., so I would be getting a late start. No big deal.

Still undecided as to which direction to run it. I drove the road and measured the mileage, leaving one liter of Gatorade between mile 4 and 5, and the next one at around mile 7, along with some water bottles at various points. I also measured the side loop, which passes by the American cannon fortifications overlooking the Hudson River. I hate this loop, as I do any loop on which you have to backtrack. It seems so long (one mile) and is all downhill, which means you have to run uphill to get back to where you started. No matter which direction I take, there is no avoiding a long uphill climb at some point. It is very demoralizing.

After parking and stretching, I was ready to run by 9:30. And I had come to a decision. My plan this time was to go against the flow of traffic, but run the uphill part first while I was fresh, saving the downhill parts for later. I was not sure what I would do when I reached the last 1¾ miles, which is mostly uphill. If I had to walk, I would.

I reached my first water bottle without a problem and drank a little less than half of it. Next came a gradual uphill, and still I felt good. I stopped at my next bottle and drank a little more. This one tasted better, probably because I was finally getting thirsty. Now to tackle the bigger hills.

I climbed the last big one, came down the other side, and took the loop. So far, so good. At the turn-around point I glanced back at that big hill. The last time I had looked at it from here, I was hurting, beaten, and dejected. Now I felt elated. I had run the entire way up without too much trouble, and had even picked up my pace a little, just so I didn't fall behind in my time. From here it was two miles back to the car. Along the way, I noticed the ½-mile marker beside a service road that connects two different sections of my route. This gave me an idea. If I ran with the traffic, then doubled back and cut through the service road, I could avoid that last big hill.

Back at the car I checked the *MapMyRun* app, which had recorded the details of the entire ten-mile run. My average speed was 5.2 miles/hour, and my time was 1 hour 56 minutes. Not great; but if it's the best I ever do, I'll take it. I changed my shirt, drank some water, took an energy gel pack, and started the second lap.

This time I ran with the flow of traffic rather than against it. Running in this direction seemed more pleasant, if only because it was new. I reached the peak of the first hill (in this direction; in the other direction, it is the last hill), and as I crested the top, what a view met my eyes: the blue, placid Hudson River and, beyond it, the foothills of Vermont's Green Mountains. Amazing what a difference a change of perspective makes. I stopped to enjoy it a few moments before continuing back down the other side of the hill. You would think running downhill would be easier than uphill, but it actually places more stress on the ankles (because of the extra force of the longer step) and thighs (from leaning backwards to maintain one's center of gravity). But it does stretch the thigh muscles, which is a good thing.

At the bottom of the hill came the loop. Time for another gel pack, and then away I went to finish the rest of the lap, which takes me back up another hill. By the time I topped the hill and reached my first water bottle, I was over 14 miles into the run and still feeling okay. After another mile or so down the road, I reached the service road at the 5¼-mile marker. I had turned off the tracking app (because it was draining my iPhone's battery), so my time and distance were estimates at best. But now I had an idea. Sure, I am able to walk and chew gum at the same time. The real question was: could I run and do math at the same time?

I calculated that if I was at mile 5¼ now and ended up at the ½-mile marker on the other side of the service road, then I would need to run just over 4 miles more on this section of the route to complete 20 miles. My mind raced with numbers. Were my calculations correct? I plodded on. I passed my last water bottle without stopping, ran another 2⅛ miles or so, and turned around. When I reached the water bottle again, I stopped and finished it, ran a little more, and then turned onto the service road, hoping that my calculations were correct. Keeping up a constant pace, I made it back to the car and checked my watch: 1 hour 58 minutes. A respectable second lap, consistent with the first. I had just completed a 20-mile run in under four hours.

I drank and rested. Nothing hurt, but I was tired. Did I have another two miles left in me at that point? Another four? Or what if…? In my heart of hearts, I believe that with more water on hand today, I could have run even further. With every succeeding workout, it seems I run about two miles more than the previous one. Twenty-six miles no longer seems like an utter impossibility. For the first time, the glimmer of hope that I can succeed has now become a bright light. I might actually be able to do this.

DAY 17
April 14 — Saratoga

I knew I would not have much free time for a full workout this weekend, so on the way home from work last night I dropped off a few bottle of water along the route I planned to run the next day. This morning I woke up, stretched, ate something, and started to run—down West Ave., followed by a loop through the state park, and then the long way back home. At 5.2 miles/hour for 1¾ hours, I ran about 10 miles today.

DAY 18
April 21 — Saratoga

My wife's car needed to go into the shop today, but I also wanted to squeeze in a long run, if possible. How to kill two birds with one stone? I know—drop off the car, then run home! Unfortunately, the dealership is near the mall. Too many cars around, which does not make for optimum running, unless I stick to side roads. So on a map of Saratoga I plotted out a one-way course that looked to be about 22–24 miles long.

Driving to the mall that morning, I traced the route in reverse, dropping off bottles of Gatorade and water along the way. One leg of the route passed through the state park, and there I left another bottle, as well as a clean shirt to change into. From here the roads got increasingly busy. As I got closer to the mall, I could see from the mileage on the odometer that I may have underestimated the distance. At that point I had two choices: take either the more direct route on a nicer road, or the longer route on a busy highway. I opted for the first choice, which turned out to be exactly 21 miles. It was a little shorter than desired (I was hoping for something closer to 23 miles), but there was less likelihood that I would be struck by a car. Or so I told myself to justify the decision.

I dropped the car off and immediately began running. Even though I was still anxious to avoid the busy highway, I knew I needed to do more than 21 miles. A voice inside me kept insisting, "If you cheat, you are only cheating yourself." No sense arguing with myself. At the last minute, I made up my mind (again) to take the longer route on the highway.

A mile down the road, I realized my ankle wasn't hurting the way it had been before. An encouraging surprise! This was the first time since God knows when that it hadn't hurt. As the day progressed, it would begin to ache a little, but nothing like before.

I reached my first series of turns and started putting distance between me and the congestion of the mall. As I approached the historic Yaddo Retreat, I decided on the spur of the moment to take a detour through its beautiful gardens. It gave me a good feeling to run some extra distance, just because I wanted to.

Outside Yaddo I was back on the busy highway, the one I had wanted to avoid. But the shoulder was wide and the sun was shining and my feet where moving, and that's all that mattered.

By the time I reached my next turn, five miles from the dealership, I was warmed up and hitting my groove. Good thing too, because now the sky was becoming overcast and the air chillier. This road traverses a ridge between two lakes, funneling the wind down the middle. It blew pretty damn hard, and I was running against it. Although I didn't feel thirsty when I reached my first water bottle, I forced myself to drink it anyway. I would need the fluids soon and did not want to get depleted beforehand.

In the state park, I felt like I had entered familiar territory. By now, my shirt was soaked with sweat, and it felt good to change into the dry one that I had left here. I was 10 miles from the mall and 13 miles from home. Still a lot of distance to cover.

The run through the park was pleasant. This is where I had done my first outdoor practice for the New Year's Eve 5K race. I passed the Victoria Pool, the Geyser spouter, and a stream where some fathers were fishing with their kids. As I started up the hill at the edge of the park, I reminded myself of what Jeff keeps telling me: "Hills make you stronger."

Outside the park I encountered another hill. The problem with the course I had mapped out is that the majority of the hills are on the second half, with most of them concentrated in the final quarter of the run. Wind and temperature were also becoming an issue. It blew so hard that I felt as if I were running against the current of a river. I was also getting cold and, to make matters worse, now the sky began to spit snow. At the next water bottle, I changed my hat, which was now very sweaty. I knew I had passed the 15-mile point, but I was tiring fast and had to push hard to keep going.

At Grand Ave. I veered left onto the loop that would bring me to the end of that road. I hate running dead-end loops. At the final turn was my last water bottle, and then another hill. The end was in sight, figuratively if not literally. Somehow I made it up the hill, reached the next water bottle, and drank deeply. Now 18 miles were behind me. Once I hit 20 miles, I would be entering new territory. The challenge excited me. I needed that now. I was looking for a kudu to chase.

I arrived at what I figured to be the 20-mile mark. From here, the usual route home would have measured a total of 21 miles. That alone would have been some kind of achievement for me. Yet, I wanted more. I needed more. I needed that psychological boost not just of passing my previous limit, but of passing it by a wide margin. So instead of taking the turn that would have brought me directly home, I kept going straight.

By now my shirt and hat were soaked through. Luckily, I had left a bandanna along this part of the route for precisely that reason. Sweat was pouring off my head and dripping into my eyes. Once again it felt good to put on something dry.

Rounding the next corner, I was greeted again by a strong wind pushing against me, but I just kept running. My pace had slowed greatly by now, and I wished for just a fraction of the strength I had had at the beginning of the run. But I had no choice but to work with what I had left in me, little as it was. I prodded myself on with this thought: *One more hill, and you're home.*

It's funny how one can drive the same road every day and not pay attention to little details. When I reached the turn at what I thought was the top of the hill, I realized that the hill kept going. To make matters worse, once I crested the actual top of the hill, I was hit head-on by a steady blast of wind. It blew hard enough to stop me dead in my tracks. Then a rumbling started in the pit of my belly, rose up through my chest, and burst from my mouth in the form of what only can be described as a primal growl. It came out in defiance of the wind, of the cold, of the snow, and in defiance of everyone who had ever told me, "You cannot." The growl came out so hard and loud that it split the wind. Putting my head down and pushing with every ounce of strength remaining in me, I stepped into that opening. I moved. I was running again.

One very long mile later, I reached the next turn of my route, taking me out of the headwind and onto the home stretch. Only half a mile more to go, and I will have run 23 miles, just three miles short of marathon distance.

Here an interesting thought entered my mind. During an actual marathon, would I be able to manage those last three miles? Maybe. And why not? It would be just like running all the way down Grand Ave. again, which I have run many times before. With the reward of a finish line in front of me, I thought I might be able to do it. Besides, if endurance was my big worry, I reminded myself that there would not be so much uphill running during the second half of the Vermont marathon. It was certainly no slam-dunk; but now it wasn't a total fantasy either.

Enough. I stopped playing mental ping-pong with my hopes and mileage calculations. For now, home and rest were within sight.

DAY 19
April 24 (Easter Sunday) — Saratoga

It has been only three days since my long run in Saratoga, but I am feeling the need to start running again. Although the weather was not predicted to be good today, I woke up early to sunny skies and mild temperature. That clinched it, I had to go. Our plans for the day were to visit Vermont and drive the marathon route. Anna would be up and ready to leave in a few hours, so I didn't have a lot of time—not even to drop off water bottles along the route. Breakfast was a hurried affair, consisting only of yogurt and a couple slices of bread.

I had a 10-mile run mapped out from one of my previous workouts that had taken me two hours to complete the last time I had done it. I would have preferred to run a little more than that— 15 miles would have been optimum—but there just wasn't enough time. So I compromised and tacked on an extra two miles. I started out at 6:10 A.M. and, at that early hour on an Easter Sunday, expected to have the road to myself. Less than five minutes later, I came upon the first of many other runners I would meet that morning. It is definitely running season here in upstate New York.

I felt strong. More importantly, I felt encouraged to know that all the hard work was paying off. Clearly there has been a big improvement in my performance over the last few weeks.

Passing the point where I usually stow my first water bottle, I realized that I did not miss it (although, in the back of my mind, I wondered if it was smart to run without drinking). I reached Grand Ave. and turned left to do the loop that I hate so much. I didn't really hate it so much today; and that steep hill at the end didn't seem so steep to me either. At the bottom of the hill, where I usually drink my last water, I felt like I didn't need it. I did have a few packs of energy gel with me, but didn't need those either. Something has changed—my endurance, for one thing. This body of mine can go longer and run more efficiently with less food and water.

Almost at the 12-mile mark. Approaching the last turn, a voice from behind startled me. It was another runner who, because she was just starting out, had a speed advantage and quickly overtook me. We chatted as we ran. One thing Jeff had stressed to me repeatedly was not to talk too much during the race, to stay focused and save my breath. I will follow this advice during the race, but for now it was pleasant having someone to talk to. I shared with her my hopes and thoughts about the upcoming adventure in Vermont, and told her about running in the battlefield. She said, "Training there is really hard because of all the hills." I just smiled. She got that right—and I was the stronger for it. We parted ways at the next intersection, and soon I arrived back home.

According to the *MapMyRun* app, I had run for 2 hours 2 minutes at a pace of 6 miles/hour. The last time, when I ran just the 10-mile part of this course, it had taken me two hours. It's not just my endurance; my speed has improved too.

I quickly showered, and then we left for Vermont to check out the course. To get to Bennington, which is about 60 miles away, one must drive through Washington County along the beautiful Battenkill River and through the rolling hills of Vermont. Upon arrival, our first order of business was to locate the hotel where we would be staying the night before the race. Next stop: the Bennington Pottery Company, the oldest pottery maker left in New England. We have several of their bowls at home. Although Anna does not share my taste or liking for the early Americana look of their products, I hoped that seeing the inside of the factory might give her a new appreciation for this style of kitchenware. A few minutes and $128 later, my plan seemingly worked all too well. Be careful what you wish for!

From there we headed over to the Arts Center, where the race would begin. Armed only with a small map printed off the Shires of Vermont Marathon website, we started to drive. After a few turns we arrived at the first landmark, Bennington Monument—an obelisk very much like the Washington Monument, except smaller. The battlefield in Saratoga has one just like it too.

An interesting historical note here. It was at the Battles of Saratoga (there were actually two of them) in 1777 that the American forces stopped the British advance, marking a crucial turning point in the Revolutionary War. Before that, however, a large contingent of Burgoyne's troops had been met by a ragtag rebel militia and defeated at the Battle of Bennington (which actually took place in Walloomsac, New York, about 10 miles away). Over 1,000 of Burgoyne's troops were wiped out, and it was this depletion of his forces that ultimately led to his surrender in Saratoga. I found it immensely fitting to discover this close historical connection between Saratoga, where I had been practicing for my first marathon, and Bennington, where I would actually be running it.

We continued driving, using the small, inadequate website map as our guide. I was surprised to learn that the middle section of the course traverses unpaved, gravel-covered roads for about five miles. Moreover, that stretch included more uphill grades than I wanted to see. I have never run on gravel before, and had no idea how I would fare on it.

Eventually we hit paved road again, which I like much better. From Arlington, where the Norman Rockwell museum used to be located before it moved to Massachusetts, we drove up the very familiar Route 7, and then on to a series of side roads, with which I was completely unfamiliar. Arriving at Hildene Meadows Park (the historic home of Robert Todd Lincoln) and the end of the course, I was elated to discover that the last five miles are fairly flat. Is it too soon to say, "Piece o' cake…"?

With all our wrong turns along the way, the 26-mile course took us 47 miles to drive. I sure hope I don't get lost during the race!

DAY 20
April 29 — Saratoga

Fifteen more days to go. If I were a horse, I would be chomping at the bit already.

Today I planned on doing one more long run of 24 miles. Everyone tells me that I should be winding down this close to race day, but I really feel the need to achieve that distance, just to prove to myself that I can do it. Besides, I will still have two weeks to rest up. Dr. Parker had advised me that to reach maximum performance, one should lay off the heavy workouts for five weeks before a big run. In the same breath, though, he added, "But if you feel like running, then run." My thought is to do a big run today, 10 miles on Monday, and another 10–15 on Friday or Saturday. After that, I will stop running completely the week before the race.

In preparation for this final big pre-race run, last evening I drove though the battlefield and left behind some water bottles and a dry shirt. This morning I woke earlier than usual, feeling very nervous about the workout. Was I doing the right thing by running so far and ignoring the advice of so many people? What if I could not complete the 24 miles? There would be no opportunity to try it again. If that happened, I would be saddled with the nagging doubt that running an entire 26-mile course might be beyond my physical capability. The last thing you want to do is question yourself. Running a marathon is 50% strength and endurance; the other 50% is psychology. I needed all 100% if I hoped to achieve my goal.

I loaded the car and drove to the battlefield. It was a beautiful spring morning, cool and clear, and the birds were out singing everywhere. I dressed, stretched, and started running. Once again, I ran against the flow of traffic so as to get the challenging hills out of the way during the first half of the workout. Of course, there were plenty of other hills to deal with in the second part.

After three miles, I saw the first of many deer. Not quite a kudu, but close enough. When I reached the first water bottle (at around four miles), I did not feel the least thirsty. I passed it by, thinking that the fluids would do me more good later in the run. I was right. At around six miles I reached the second water bottle, and this time I drank, because I needed to. I was learning to listen to my body.

Next came the dreaded loop, but now it didn't bother me. I knew it would get harder soon, but for now I was actually enjoying myself.

From the end of the loop to the top of the hill is a mile. That was not bad either. At about the 8½-mile mark, my legs began to go slower, but I still wasn't tired. Once I made it to the car, I would drink some Gatorade, which would refuel me with 200 calories. *Maybe I shouldn't wait that long.* It was too early in the game to fall behind in the energy department, so I ate an energy gel. What a difference that made. Within a half mile, I felt reinvigorated and reached the car in good time. I had done 10 miles in 2 hours—not bad for me. I changed my shirt, drank a liter of Gatorade, and began my second lap.

At the top of the big hill I kept running, but made sure to look up and take in the view. You can see all the way to Vermont. The route I had chosen would bring me back to this same spot at mile 22. I told myself, *When you see this view again, then you'll know that you can run a marathon.*

On the other side of the hill, I came again to the dreaded loop, which I didn't mind this time either; but when I started up the long hill in the other direction, I began to tire. Cresting that hill, I arrived at my next water bottle. The first time I had passed this way, I drank half of it; this time I finished it off.

I ran down the road a little more and encountered another good-sized hill. Jeez, this place is uphill in both directions. *Time for another energy gel pack.*

Approaching the mile-5 marker and the service road that would bring to the return stretch, I began to tire out, but the miles were clicking away. I paused at the water bottle I had ignored on my first pass, drank half of it, and kept going. The place where the British forces had their headquarters was my turn-around point. I was glad to see it. For the British, it symbolized defeat; for me, victory. After this, I would be on the home stretch.

Here I ate another gel pack for the energy boost, which I sorely needed at this point. Next I found and finished my bottle of Gatorade, and then headed for the service road. I felt pretty whipped by now, but was cheered by the thought of the dry shirt waiting for me there. I changed but did not drink anything, allowing myself the respite of walking the 50 yards to the next section of road. Then I began running again, all the way to the top of the hill in front of me.

Yes, *that* hill. Mile 22. Below me flowed the Hudson and, looming in the distance, Vermont. *When you see this view again, then you'll know you can run a marathon.* So now I knew. I was convinced, without a doubt, that I could run the entire 26 miles.

From here I would have to get back to the car one way or another, and I was determined that I would do it running. What better way to celebrate this breakthrough?

I started back, first downhill, then uphill, followed by even more uphills after that, plugging away for all I was worth. I had to slow down for the last couple of miles, but was still running by the time I had completed the full 24-mile course. If I had taken another gel pack, I am absolutely certain I could have run—yes, *run*—another two miles, but decided against it. I had accomplished what I had set out to do today, and that made me happy. Besides, I had better things to eat in the car. I just need to remember not to short myself on gel packs the day of the race.

At last, the killer runs are behind me now. Well, at least for the next two weeks.

DAY 21
May 1 — Saratoga

My body felt very tight and stiff the day after my long run. The next day, though, it felt much better. Today I tried a short workout of 7 miles, just to see how I would do. It was enjoyable not having to push myself through a killer run.

DAY 22
May 6 — Saratoga

I should be resting this week, restricting myself to short runs. My plan initially was to do just 10 miles today but decided to do more, mapping out an ambitious 14–15-mile route. Starting out, I felt good and loose; but nearing the 10-mile mark, my legs tightened up, with no sign that they would get loose again anytime soon. So I called it a day. The legs didn't really hurt at all, but I certainly was not running at peak speed. I think I could have gone the distance, had I tried, but it would not have been pretty.

DAY 23
May 9 — Saratoga

My last training run. I drove to the state park with the intention of running only 5 miles. Once again, though, something compelled me to do more, so instead I ran about 9 miles. It just felt good to be running. My leg muscles were loose and relaxed. I hope I feel this good the day of the race.

I bought myself a new Dry-Plus shirt and wore it for the first time today. I certainly did sweat a lot less while running. Whether it was due to the wind or the cooler temperatures, or maybe the shirt itself, I'm not sure. Perhaps I won't need to change my shirt three times during the race!

I got home and took off my running shoes, saying to myself, *The next time you take off these shoes, you will be a marathon runner.*

CHAPTER 4

The Race

The day before the race, we packed and drove to Bennington, arriving early. I dropped Anna off at a belly dance workshop (an art form at which she has become quite adept, much to my delight), while I went to Marathon headquarters to pick up the racing packet with my number, electronic timer, and other supplies. While there, I wandered through an exhibition of running clothes and shoes on display, along with Vermont-made products like cheese, maple syrup, and some very tasty maple cookies.

For those of you who have never had real maple syrup, you don't know what you are missing. My wife and I travel throughout Vermont every spring, stopping at the sugarhouses where they boil the sap into syrup, releasing great billows of steam into the air. It takes 32 to 40 quarts of sap to make one quart of syrup. That's a lot of steam! The room with the evaporator is engulfed in a thick mist of the stuff, just like a sauna, except for the pungently sweet aroma of maple sugar delighting the nostrils. If you have never experienced a sugarhouse in action, you should really put it on your bucket list.

Before leaving to pick up Anna from the belly dance studio, I stopped by the tourist information desk to get some recommendations for restaurants in the area. I had been carbo-loading for the past few days at home, and I was looking forward to a tasty meal out.

Around dinnertime, it began to rain. We had decided to try an eating spot that was supposed to be a favorite of the locals, at least according to the lady at the tourist information desk. Apparently she was telling the truth, because it looked like the entire populace of Bennington had descended upon the place all at once. A line of hungry customers snaked out the door and into the parking lot. We were told that it would be a 45-minute wait before we could be seated. I was starting to get the pre-race jitters, and I wasn't sure that I could even sit through dinner for that length of time, let alone stand in the rain just waiting to eat.

Right down the street we noticed another restaurant that looked much less busy, so we thought we'd give that a shot instead. It was an old building that appeared to have once been a private residence, now renovated into an intimate bistro-style eatery.

Walking in, we saw at once that it not only lacked crowds, it lacked customers. The place was practically empty. *Uh-oh, not a good sign.* I said to Anna, "What do the locals know that we don't?"

At least getting seated wouldn't be a problem. And besides, all I wanted to eat was pasta. How bad could they screw that up? As it turned out, the food was excellent, but it was hard for me to enjoy it. Any other night I would have welcomed the leisurely meal—but not that night. I was too antsy. Sitting there and listening to the rain outside while my mind raced full speed ahead, I could not get myself to relax. A glass of wine might have helped, but all the training manuals I had read advised limiting alcohol consumption the night before a marathon. (Besides, I was saving my "alcohol ration" for later that night, in case I had trouble sleeping.) Finally, after I asked my wife twice if she wanted to take the rest of her food to the hotel and finish it there, I realized I had to stop worrying so much. At the time, I could not say for sure what I was worried about. Only later, when a few weeks had passed, did it occur to me that it was the rain that had me so spooked. I had thought about this day a thousand times in a thousand ways—what could go wrong, what could go right—but not once did I think of rain. It was the one variable I had not anticipated.

I paid the bill and we headed back to the hotel. While Anna took a shower, I organized my running clothes and watched the weather channel. Then I reorganized my running clothes and watched the weather channel some more. After several repetitions of this routine, the weather outlook remained the same, my clothes were back in their original piles, and I was no closer to relaxing.

After a while, I took half an Ambien, washed down with a small glass of Grand Marnier. Several weather reports later, somewhere around 10:00 P.M., my brain finally shut down and my eyes closed in sleep to the sound of falling rain.

೦૨ɛഠ

At six in the morning I woke up abruptly. Something seemed different. It was too quiet. No rain! Maybe the weatherman was wrong. Gee, that never happens, does it? I quietly rolled out of bed, put on my warm-up clothes (which, just for the record, I had finally managed to get organized and nicely laid out), and went downstairs.

Looking outside, I could see the parking lot dotted with puddles, but nary a raindrop in sight. The dark clouds overhead were thinning out, with a promising brightness starting to filter though. I brought a cup of coffee with me into the exercise room, surprised to find myself alone there. Surely I was not the only person who had trouble sleeping the morning of a race.

One of my leg muscles was causing me some concern. I thought it might not loosen up in time. If it started to go into spasms during the race, I would not be able to finish. Every time I looked down at the leg, I could see the muscle quivering, the same way it did at the 14-mile point on my first run through the battlefield weeks before. I dreaded that thought and was determined not to let it happen. I began my stretching routine, bracing my foot against something about knee-high and leaning into it. I could feel the muscle contract, stay tight, and then begin to loosen. Next I worked on the other leg. Then I lifted the foot higher and repeated the stretching exercise. Soon I had my leg up as high as my hip. So far, so good. After that, I methodically worked all my muscle groups, arms, shoulders, back. Now it was time to meet the day.

I knew I should be drinking a moderate amount of fluids, but coffee was not the best choice. Still, I had one more cup. I sat and talked with the man at the front desk. He said the rain was definitely coming. I hoped that he was wrong, or that at least it would come late in the day. I had been up for an hour by now, and still I did not see another runner. How could they all be sleeping so late? Weren't they too excited to sleep, too nervous, too scared?

Back in the room, I filled Anna in on my morning so far while she dressed. Then I showered, we packed most of our things, and headed down for breakfast. I already knew what I wanted: waffles. I had cut them out when I was on my diet, but now I was supposed to be carbo-loading, so they were fair game. Once we sat down, however, it dawned on me that I wasn't really all that hungry. My mind was elsewhere. We ate a quiet breakfast, talking only to go over final plans. By this time we had already gone over those final plans twenty times, but it was all I could think or talk about.

With breakfast over, it was time to get the show on the road.

I had several piles of clothes laid out on the bed—shorts, socks, toecaps, and running shoes in one pile, and three shirts and three hats in the other. If it rained, the hats would come in handy.

I sweat a lot when I run. During training, my shirts would get so drenched and uncomfortable that I would have to change to a dry one every ten miles. For that reason, I arranged for Anna to meet me twice along the course, once at 8 miles and again at 20 miles, so I could change my shirt and hat.

I made one small mistake in the matter of the shirts, a mistake that would come back to haunt me later in the race. Up until the last few weeks, all my training runs were done early in the morning in the late winter and early spring, when the temperature was typically cool, if not downright cold. I always wore a long-sleeved shirt. As the weather warmed up, however, I needed something lighter. All they sold at the local running store was clothing made from the dry-tech synthetic fabric. As soon as I felt how light and soft they were, I ditched the old cotton shirts and bought three of the newfangled ones to wear for this race. And that's where I made my mistake.

These shirts were the only items of clothing I had not worn at least once during my training runs. One of the first things I ever read about running a marathon stated that you should never try anything new during a race. *Wear what you trained in.* That small but important rule of thumb had completely slipped my mind.

We checked out and drove directly to the Arts Center, the starting point of the race. The building is nestled against the side of a tree-covered hill. The rain from the day before made the leaves appear crisper and greener than usual. Thin, wispy clouds shrouded the tops of the surrounding hills. Then a misty rain began to fall, very light at first, almost unnoticeable. All around we saw runners in various stages of preparation. Some were stretching, some were jogging, and still others were pinning racing numbers on themselves. I didn't know any of them, but I felt a special camaraderie with all of them. I knew many had run marathons before and had already secured their standing as marathon runners. I was not in their league yet, but felt I had earned the right to stand and run among them. I had put in the work and time, had run the distances, and proudly bore the battle scars: the black and blue toes, the sore knees, the pulled muscles. No, I was not one of them yet, but I deserved to be there as much as anyone.

I pulled both my knee braces into place and put on my shoes, thinking again that the next time I took them off, I would be a marathon runner.

We walked around, soaking in all the sights and sounds. The atmosphere was electric, but I felt only restlessness and apprehension. We tried to take in some of the artwork on display, but the center was too crowded, and my heart was just not in it. Outside, the mist had become a light rain. I wanted to warm up but did not want to expend energy running, so we just walked. I posed for a picture under the starting banner.

About then it struck me: *This is for real.* My work, my dreams, my determination, they all came down to this. Not a single day had passed in the last six months that I did not spend all my free time thinking about what was about to take place. Right then and there, I told Anna something I had never told anyone else before. I told her that I always knew, even when I was at my fattest, that one day I would run a marathon.

According to the schedule, handicapped racers would start at 9:00 A.M.; and then at 9:10 the rest of the runners would go. The handicapped racers, about ten of them, were paraplegics who had lost the use of their legs. Each one sat strapped into a handbike, which looks similar to a regular bicycle, except it has three wheels and is lower to the ground. Instead of using foot pedals, the runners move by turning hand pedals on a bar between their legs. I admired them and felt humbled. Here I was, patting myself on the back for all that I had overcome to get to this point; yet all my efforts could not hold a candle to what any of these men and women had had to face.

Starting time drew near. I went over the meeting spots one more time with Anna and said my goodbyes. She jockeyed herself into position on the sidelines for photographs. Anyone who does long-distance running will tell you that it is a lonely sport. Although I was standing in the middle of a crowd of three hundred and fifty people, never before have I felt so alone. It did not matter. I knew what was going to happen next. I knew what had to be done. I was totally focused on one thing, and one thing only. I was ready.

ଔଛୀ

At 9:00 A.M. sharp, the handicapped riders started. Within the first 50 yards, they hit speeds that staggered me. They were followed by a cadre of motorcyclists, whose job it was to monitor them and offer help, but I doubted any of them would need it. In fact, the motorcyclists would have trouble keeping up with them!

I made my way toward the front of the crowd of runners, positioning myself to get the best time possible. I certainly did not want to be in the front row; that was for the advanced runners. But at least I wasn't at the tail end of the pack. Then at 9:10 precisely, the starting gun fired, and I took my first step on one of the biggest adventures of my life.

Like a flock of birds taking wing, the runners moved forward, slowly at first, because we were all crowded so close together, but then gaining speed as we spread out across the length and breadth of the road. I was on the right side of the pack. Anna was on the left somewhere, so I edged my way toward the other side, taking care not to get in the way of other runners. My eyes scoured the crowd of onlookers and well-wishers, to no avail. I thought I may have run past her already, but then suddenly I spotted her. She was videotaping the start of the marathon. I came up close to blow her a kiss as I passed by, which I now do habitually at every race now. This gesture has become my good luck talisman.

En masse, the pack of runners rounded a bend in the road and headed toward the Bennington Monument. For me, running again after a two-week hiatus felt very comfortable, like visiting an old friend. Taking the left turn at the monument, I was amazed at how good this felt, how much I wanted to move fast. In the excitement of the race, it is easy to start too strong, and then you will tire out early. I thought of the story Jeff told me about his first marathon. He was running strong and passed some old-timer, who told him, "Slow up, buddy, you have a long way to go." Jeff didn't listen and raced far ahead. Later in the race, the old-timer caught up with Jeff, easily passed him, and left him in the dust. So I tried to pace myself right from the get-go. I didn't much care who passed me; I just didn't want to poop out too early. With Jeff's story knocking around in my head, I picked out another runner, an older man who looked like he had experience, and who was running at about my speed. I decided to match my pace to his.

It was fun watching the different runners and their styles. One young man, in his mid-twenties and in shape, I remember in particular. He ran like a gazelle. His stride was a kind of bounding bounce, with both feet off the ground at the same time, yet each leg moving independently of the other.

At the bottom of the first long hill, the route ran along a pretty little river. Most of the rivers in Vermont are "freestone streams." These consist of fast-moving water that flows over rocks and around boulders. The water in these rivers is usually gin-clear, but the recent rains had turned this one muddy and brown. I did make a mental note to come back and fish it someday.

I was still fifty feet behind my pacer, and doing well despite the light rain. Somewhere in the distance, I could hear the unmistakable sound of bagpipes. Directly ahead was a covered bridge—something else (besides cheese and maple syrup) that

Vermont is famous for. Standing just inside the bridge, away from the rain, was a bagpiper. Pretty cool. It made me feel special

On the other side of the bridge I came to the first water station—and ran right by it. I was so busy thinking about the piper that I forgot about the water. I certainly did not need to drink yet, but I did not want to get dehydrated either. Thoughts of my quivering thigh kept popping into my head. I would be sure to drink at the next stop.

Ahead of me, at the entrance to Bennington College, loomed the first real hill of the course. The hill was long and curved to the left. It went up, as hills tend to do; but so did I. The pack began to thin out by now. I was starting to recognize the people around me. Some of them I had passed once already, and then they had passed me back. We would do this all day long.

In North Bennington, the town where Anna and I had dined the night before, I grabbed a cup at the water station and drank on the run. Not too far up the road, I knew Anna would be waiting for me.

Just outside the village, one of my fellow runners, a young guy, came up alongside me and asked, "Are you an old marine type guy?" I replied, "No, just an old type guy." I took the remark as a compliment, and told him about my A-fib and about my new diet and about the subsequent weight loss. He said I should definitely get the award for "most improved." Then Jeff's words came back to me again. He had told me that people were going to want to talk with me. "Don't do it," he said. "Not on your first marathon. Save your breath to save your strength." His advice was usually spot-on, so I deliberately slowed down and let the amiable talker pass ahead of me.

The gentle morning mist, which earlier had turned into a light drizzle, had become a steady rain by now. My original plan was to meet Anna at several points along the way and change my shirts, which I knew would be heavy with sweat. At this point the plan no longer made any practical sense. Sure, I was drenched, but more from the rain than from sweating. It wouldn't matter how often I changed; the shirts would just get wet again.

The night before, I had chosen a spot at the eight-mile mark with adequate parking and marked it on the GPS, so Anna would have no trouble finding it. As I approached the spot, I realized that other people had had the same idea. The area was crawling with cars, and I thought we might not be able to find each other in the crowd. If I missed her, I hoped she wouldn't worry about me.

Yet there she was, standing in the rain, taking my picture with a camera. She asked how I was and if I needed anything. Tossing my wet hat into open hatchback, I grabbed a dry one and told her I was fine and would see her at the next stop. A quick kiss, and I was off and running again. I felt a little sorry for Anna. At least I was doing something. She, on the other hand, had sat there in the rain for an hour waiting for me. That had to be boring. But as she would tell me later, it was fun for her to be part of the excitement.

A few miles later, I reached the middle section of the course. Here it turned onto what Vermonters endearingly like to call "rural roads." By that they mean unpaved dirt roads. Many people prefer running on unpaved roads, because they think it is easier on the knees. Perhaps it is, although some recent studies suggest otherwise. For me, the potholes proved to be a distraction. I run most effectively when I settle into a rhythm; and in order to avoid the potholes, I was forced to change my stride. "A hole is just a hole," you say? Not when the hole is full of muddy water. Even though my running shoes were now well worn, I instinctively did not want to get them dirty. Blame it on my mother, who had a "thing" about dirt.

It was hard to keep up with the older gentleman by whom I was trying to set my own pace. Because he was obviously experienced, I knew it was inevitable that I would fall far behind him sooner or later, even though we were running at more or less the same speed. After my rendezvous with Anna, I lost sight of him completely, but knew he could not be too far away. I picked up my pace until he came into view again, a good hundred yards in front of me and moving at a solid, steady pace. Even from that far away, I could tell that he knew what he was doing and how to stay in control. As much as I wanted to catch up to him, that ambition proved futile. I was slowing and he was not. About then nature called and I ran into the bushes to pee. That was the last I saw of him.

Now I was entering hill territory. I was not at all worried, though, because I had trained on hills a lot in Saratoga. As Jeff always said, "Hills make you stronger." He was right, and I felt confident that I could handle whatever was in store. Any marathon runner will tell you that it's not your legs that make you win, it's your head. So self-confidence was one thing I had going for me— possibly the most important thing.

Between miles 10 and 15, the route tracked mostly uphill. Few of the hills were killers, but they were hills nevertheless, intermingled with a series of level plateaus. By now I had joined up with a group of other runners. A surprising number of them stopped and took the hills at a brisk walk. That is when I left a lot of them behind. I figured they would catch up to me again eventually, and probably pass by me. Frankly, I didn't much care who was in front. My only goal was to finish the race.

Even though I still felt strong, my legs were beginning to tighten up. This concerned me. I knew that if I slowed to a walk, it would be impossible for me to start running again. I would never be able to finish the race. As long as there was breath in my body, that simply was not an option. So I kept on running.

The road here was barely two lanes wide, with trees growing close to the shoulders. The thick, green foliage limited visibility in most areas; but on one short stretch the trees opened up, revealing a gorgeous vista to the left. The hill dropped off sharply into a large meadow with a stream meandering through it and a bog in the middle. The hills on the other side were shrouded in hazy clouds. It looked like something out of *National Geographic*. All that was missing from the scene was a moose (or a kudu). It took all my concentration to make it up the hill, so I could not enjoy the view as much as I would have liked. It was gone as quickly as it came.

I spent a lot of time looking down at the ground in front of me. When you do that, you see many things that would ordinarily be missed. The rain had brought out the earthworms en masse. Their slimy, slithery bodies littered the ground. As much as I did not want to break my stride, I tried to avoid stepping on them so as to spare their lives. I also noticed a lot of dead frogs. I think most had been run over by cars the night before, because they looked pretty flat.

The halfway point of the race was a welcome sight indeed. It came out of nowhere in the midst of a heavy downpour. The volunteers were out in force, handing out water and energy gel packs at a furious rate. I needed both now. I grabbed a cup of water first and washed that down with some Gatorade. Next I ate a gel pack, keeping an extra one for later.

My kudu was on the run, and still out of reach. But I was closing in on my prey.

Finally the hills began to level off, and I was grateful to hit pavement again. It was still raining heavily when I approached the 16-mile mark, smack-dab in the middle of a large dairy farm surrounded by green pastures, made greener still by the rain. I passed a white barn with an irrigation pond beside it. Glancing up, I noticed a photographer kneeling by the roadside and his assistant holding an umbrella. His camera was pointed directly at me. I gave him the biggest smile I could muster. In the picture, which he showed me later, the photographer had framed me perfectly with the barn in the background. That is my favorite photograph from the race.

By the time I came to the next water station, I had lost track of the mileage. I drank my water and Gatorade and asked one of the ladies at the station, "Am I at mile 19 yet?" She replied, almost apologetically, "No, this is only mile 17." I think her answer bothered her more than me. As it turns out, my favorite stretch of any marathon I have run usually occurs between the 15- and 20- mile marks. Whenever I talk about running with anyone, I like to say that the first ten miles are fun. Over the next five miles, though, I start to think, *This isn't so much fun.* Sometime after that, when I've covered a full fifteen miles, the running becomes work—but it's the kind of work I like. I feel as though I have truly accomplished something. And that is when the endorphins, the brain's own natural mood-enhancing and stress-relieving opiate, really start to kick in. No wonder I like this part of the race so much!

I really needed those endorphins right about now, because it was at this point that my left nipple began to get sore. I experienced this before, after my previous training runs over twenty miles. The sweaty shirt rubs against the skin and irritates it. I thought to myself, *But it's kind of early for this to be happening now.* I tried to hold my shirt away from the nipple as much as possible, but to no avail. I needed both arms swinging to maintain my rhythm, so I had little choice but to grin and bear it.

This is the small mistake I mentioned at the beginning of this chapter. I was wearing one of those new shirts that I had never run with before. Now that it had gotten wet and heavy, it rubbed against my skin more than the cotton shirts. I remembered that rule of thumb I had read about early on: *Wear what you trained in.* In other words, never try anything new the day of the race. Lesson learned.

A short way further up, I spotted a lone Vermont State Trooper cheerfully directing traffic for the runners crossing the main highway. I'm sure he had better things to do than stand in the rain all day. The sight of him doing his job without complaint gave me a deep appreciation for all the volunteers who make it possible for people like me to run.

On the approach to the village of West Arlington, I passed a street sign that read "Ice Pond Road," and wondered how the road had gotten its name. Maybe there was a pond at the end of it. I pictured a scene from long ago, something out of a faded sepia photograph: a crew of laborers standing on the frozen pond with long saws cutting out blocks of ice. Once upon a time, in the days before electric refrigeration, theirs was a very important job. The ice, insulated with straw, would be stored in large barns and stay frozen right through the summer, so that it could be used to preserve food in people's "ice boxes." I wished I could stand inside one of those ice barns right now, feeling the cool air caress my sweaty skin.

I entered the village—another welcome sight. Anna would be waiting for me at the 20-mile mark. Here, we runners were met by a crowd of onlookers along the sidelines cheering us on. Among them was a group of girls I had seen before, at the very start of the race (they were easy to recognize—one of them had purple hair). They had taken the trouble to drive from Bennington to West Arlington, despite the pouring rain, just to welcome the runners and encourage us to keep our spirits up through this last difficult leg of the marathon. I was getting very tired now; and the idea that complete strangers would care so much about the outcome of a race and the well-being of the runners helped to reinvigorate me. Indeed, at this point I came upon a long curve in the road, and I could have spared myself a good 50 yards of running by transecting the curve in a straight line. I refused to do so. Instead, I deliberately hugged the sidewalk, so that no one (least of all myself) could say I had failed to run the entire distance.

West Arlington is one of my favorite towns in Vermont. The village's picturesque Main Street is lined with big old Victorian houses, most of which have been converted to country inns and B&Bs. It's so quaint that visiting here is like stepping onto the set of *The Bob Newhart Show*. Fittingly, the Norman Rockwell Museum used to be located here before it moved across the border into Massachusetts.

It was pouring now, the rain falling heavier than it had fallen all day. Against all odds, I spotted Anna right away, standing in the deluge taking pictures. What a trooper! Unfortunately, the camera got so wet that it stopped working properly. The last photo she took was nothing but a blur.

When I reached the car, she took one look at me and said, "You're bleeding." Sure enough, the irritation around my left nipple had turned into a lesion, and blood was soaking through the shirt. It looked a little as if my chest had burst open right over the heart. Luckily, I had brought along a first-aid kit (which should be a part of every runner's arsenal of crucial accessories). Anna stuck a band aide over the nipple. On my wet skin, it didn't look like it would stay in place for long, so she applied four more band-aids around the first. Then she mentioned that the girls she had belly danced with the day before were just up the road, dancing on someone's porch. That was something to look forward to! I changed into a dry shirt, which felt good on my skin, though I knew it wouldn't stay dry for long in this weather. Then she gave me a kiss, and I said, "The next time you kiss me, you will be kissing a marathon runner." With that, I turned and started running again.

I hadn't gone far when I began to hear the exotic strains of belly dancing music, and soon I spotted the performers: a half dozen shapely women dressed in colorful, beaded outfits, swaying and shimmying in the tight confines of the porch. All of Main Street had a fun, noisy, carnival atmosphere that I regretted leaving behind. Soon I turned onto a side road that was less busy, and where the sound of belly dancing music was replaced by the drone of bagpipes. It was the same player I had first seen at the covered bridge.

Soon I arrived at the 21-mile water station, which was situated at the base of a hill. The small spurt of energy I got from my stop with Anna had begun to fade, but I gathered my strength and ran up the hill. My reward for making it to the top was a nice view of the wetlands surrounding the Battenkill River. I couldn't actually see the river itself, just the alders and willows lining the marshland along its course.

At the end of this road I faced one more small incline, and then five miles of flat running. I poured myself into that last little hill. At the top, a volunteer directing traffic turned to me and said, "Looking strong!" I thought, *Yeah, right.* I felt anything but strong.

Now I was running on a fairly flat road, which crossed over the Battenkill and made its way toward Hildene Meadows in Manchester. This has to be one of the loveliest places in the country. It is also the home of the Orvis flagship store. Here you can learn to fly fish on the banks of the Battenkill. You enter the town on Route 7, which is lined with one impressive Victorian mansion after another, each one larger than the last. In the center of town is the Equinox, a three-story hotel built in the 1800s with an elegant white porch outfitted with comfy rocking chairs. Massive maple trees, which turn brilliant orange and red and yellow in the autumn, adorn the streets. We visit this place every year just to sit on this porch and relax. This is the reason I wanted to run this race. I just love the area.

After Abraham Lincoln was assassinated, his oldest son Robert Todd Lincoln moved to Manchester and purchased what would later become known as the Hildene Estate. Now it is an historic landmark open to the public. Behind the estate lies the town's recreational area, called Hildene Meadows, which is equipped with soccer and baseball fields. The marathon's finish line is located here too. But that was still five miles away.

By now I was running on empty. I was thankful for having put in the time to do several training runs of over twenty miles. Had I not, severe (if not fatal) doubt would likely have crept in. I have since come to learn that such doubt can afflict even the most experienced runners at this part of the course. Ahead of me lay a long, tough section. Though I did not feel discouraged, I had no idea how I would manage to complete the next few miles. I liken it to childbirth: it is painful and unpleasant. But once begun, there is no going back.

During this time, a few of my fellow runners would catch up and then pass me while going at a pretty good pace. The idea that people could run faster than I did not come as any surprise to me. What I did not understand was: Why? If they could still run at that speed after twenty-two miles, why hadn't they passed me sooner? It was a mystery to me. With the exception of those few, the rest of us had long since fallen into place along the route and rarely shifted far from it.

How tired was I? From the sound of footsteps and heavy breathing, I knew there was someone not far behind me. But at this point, I had so little energy left that I did not want to waste it by turning my head to look at him.

I remember passing a house on the left. The yard was bordered with spring flowers and, behind the daffodils, a barking dog. He ran back and forth, back and forth, yapping at us as we passed by. His tail was wagging, so he was probably just happy and excited to see us. But I thought, *If he comes after me, I'm dead meat.* There is no way I could run away. Perhaps it was just mental exhaustion that made me notice these things and have such odd thoughts.

At the 24-mile mark I entered into brand new territory. I had never run this far before. I knew the end was near, but at this stage of exhaustion, two miles might as well have been a hundred. Another ten minutes passed, and I thought I could hear some commotion in the distance. What was it? Yes, no doubt: it was the sound of cheering people, emanating from a direction about 45° to the right. But I couldn't see anyone, so I figured there must be a bend in the road somewhere ahead.

The 25-mile marker drifted past, and the cheers grew louder. Among the cheers I could also hear the sound of cowbells, which many spectators at marathons bring with them to ring as the runners pass the finish line. The rain had stopped a few minutes before, and water and sweat evaporated off my skin, which now sported goose bumps. I had just run twenty-five miles, and only now was I beginning to get chilly. Go figure.

It's funny—the things you pay attention to at a moment like this. Following the sound of cheering people filtering through the line of trees, I could almost see the parking lot now. That should have been my main focus. But all I can really remember noticing is the plastic water bottle lying in a ditch. The old stone wall running at an angle up a nearby hill. The maple saplings growing alongside the wall. I remember the thud of my feet on pavement, the moistness of the air, the leaves glimmering with wetness. All my senses were attuned to what was immediately before and around me, in a rapid a sequence of ephemeral sensations that left behind indelible memories.

Rounding the last bend in the road, at last I could see people in front of me who were not runners. The onlookers lined the edge of the parking lot, some standing behind the stone fence, others sitting cross-legged on it, all cheering and shouting encouragement. I tried to run faster for them, but simply could not. I looked for Anna, my eyes scanning the crowd until they picked her out from among hundreds of happy, grinning faces. Of all the things I won't forget from that day, the most unforgettable was the expression on her face. She looked so proud of me, prouder even than I felt.

Lines of orange traffic cones guided me to the last turn. I had done it, I had run 26 miles. Yet the race was *still* not over. The official standard length of a marathon course is actually 26.2 miles. This standard was established during the 1908 Olympiad in London, when the course was slightly lengthened by 385 yards so that the runners would finish right in front of King Edward VII sitting in the Royal Box. In order for the Shires course to equal 26.2 miles, the organizers decreed that race participants must turn into the parking lot and then run the last two tenths of a mile toward the finish line, which was in the opposite direction from which they just came.

I made my turn in the fields and began that last 385-yard run back toward the official end of the course. This was the only time during the entire race that I knew for an absolute certainty that I would complete it. My eyes filled up with tears. I can't begin to tell you all the thoughts that raced through my mind at this moment. I thought of my mother who died 30 years ago, of the time after my daughter was born that I first tried to take up running, of the skunk cabbages I used to pass on my morning workouts, of my leg quivering at the 14-mile mark of my first long run. These and a thousand other thoughts passed through my mind within mere seconds.

I remember that the fields around me were filled with yellow dandelions. The banner at the finish line grew larger as I drew closer. I pushed hard to increase my speed and end in a sprint, but my legs refused move any faster. They did not need to. They had done their job that day, and that was all I could ask.

I stepped past the timing pad. It was done. I had caught my kudu. I looked for Anna, but then someone on the loudspeaker called my name, and a girl put a medal around my neck. Finally, I caught sight of my wife taking pictures of me with my iPhone. Her camera had gotten wet and shorted out, and the lens of her iPhone had fogged up. Now she was using mine. I hugged Anna, telling her breathlessly over and over again, "I did it, I did it." She said, "Yes, you did." What else could she say, or I say? These phrases, simple as they were, meant the entire world to me in those few seconds of triumph.

My official time was 5 hours and 22 minutes. By many people's standards, this was nothing to brag about, but to me it was fantastic—the fulfillment of a lifelong dream! My only goal had been merely to finish the race, and I had accomplished that. I did not race against the clock or the other runners. I raced against my past, and against all my frail human limitations. And I had won.

Although I was beyond tired, I found it all but impossible to keep still. My legs were used to moving now. Despite the lactic acid build-up and the pain and the dehydration, they just wanted to move. I walked around a bit, catching my breath and letting the muscles cool off slowly, which is much better for you than sitting down right away. Runners were still crossing the finish line. I would not have cared if I had come in dead last. But considering that this was my first marathon, it was still nice to know that mine was not the slowest time.

We popped inside the refreshment tent they had set up for the runners to see if there was anything good left for me to eat. I could have eaten whatever I wanted, but all the bananas, bagels, pizza, and cookies were already gone, and nothing else looked appetizing. I should have been starving by now, but my stomach was still upset from the energy gels. This is a common occurrence. The energy gels themselves are not the culprit; rather, during a prolonged physical workout, blood is diverted from the gut to the muscles, so anything in one's stomach just sits there, undigested. Then I caught sight of the ice cream: two large boxes, one chocolate, the other vanilla. For some reason, those appealed to me, even though they had been sitting out on a table unrefrigerated and had gotten very soft. I scooped some into a cup, grabbed a spoon, and headed toward the car.

Sitting under the hatchback and slowly eating the ice cream, I suddenly started to shake and tremble. My lips and fingernails turned blue. Hypothermia was setting in, and my core temperature was dropping rapidly. Another lesson learned: after a marathon, get out of your wet clothes right away.

Anna started the car, turned on the heat full blast, and ran back to the tent to get me a cup of hot coffee. Meanwhile, I discreetly slipped off my drenched running clothes and changed into a dry shirt, sweatpants, and socks. Then I positioned my body directly in front of the vents and let the hot air warm me up.

My legs began stiffening up worse than I have ever experienced before, so Anna drove us back home. The celebratory call to Jeff could not wait for the end of the hour-long drive, so I called him from the car. We talked like a couple of high school kids whose team has just won the state championship. That evening, while we conversed in the car, my friend and running mentor at last welcomed me into his club—that very exclusive club where the membership dues are high, but the rewards last a lifetime.

CHAPTER 5

A Johnnie Walker Blue Night

It had been several hours since our return home. All the wet clothes were unpacked and washed, all the appropriate phone calls had been made. My stiff muscles began to relax. My legs hurt a little when I stood—but it was a good hurt, the kind that comes only from pushing oneself to the limit.

Anna and I sat together on the couch and turned on the TV. Today was my day, so she let me have the controller and did not complain when I flipped through the channels. Whenever we talked (which was often), I found myself directing the conversation back to the race. I told her the same stories over and over. She listened politely, as if she had never heard them before. Did I mention? Anna is the best wife any man could wish for.

I wanted to cap off the day in a fitting manner. Years before, I had bought a small bottle of expensive Johnnie Walker Blue scotch.

It still sat in the cupboard, unopened, waiting for the right occasion to drink it. I had considered cracking it open the night after we hiked to Lake Tear of the Clouds, but now I was glad I had not.

Today was the right occasion.

You don't pour a good whiskey like this into just any old glass. Several years ago, we received a stunning set of crystal scotch glasses from Nova Scotia Crystal as a Christmas present. I took one out of the china cabinet, tossed in a couple of ice cubes, and then broke the seal on the bottle. A sweet peaty aroma filled my nostrils. The ice made popping noises as I poured the amber liquid into the glass. I swirled it around and gave it a sip. It tasted smooth, rich, and mellow. I had waited years to try this particular scotch, but it was worth the wait. I could not imagine a more perfect finish to this most prefect day.

As I sat there, quietly sipping my drink, I thought back to all the events of my life that had brought me to this moment of sweet victory. I thought of my leg quivering in the cold, of growling at the wind, of the endless hours spent wondering if I could indeed run a marathon, of the gallons of sweat I had poured into achieving my goal. I thought of the endless patience Anna had with me, and of the freedom she had given me to train. I thought of how lucky I was to have a good friend like Jeff. But mostly I thought of how lucky I was to have a dream for so many years and then to finally to have made it come true.

It is not every day that one's dreams come true. I am indeed a blessed man.

THE END

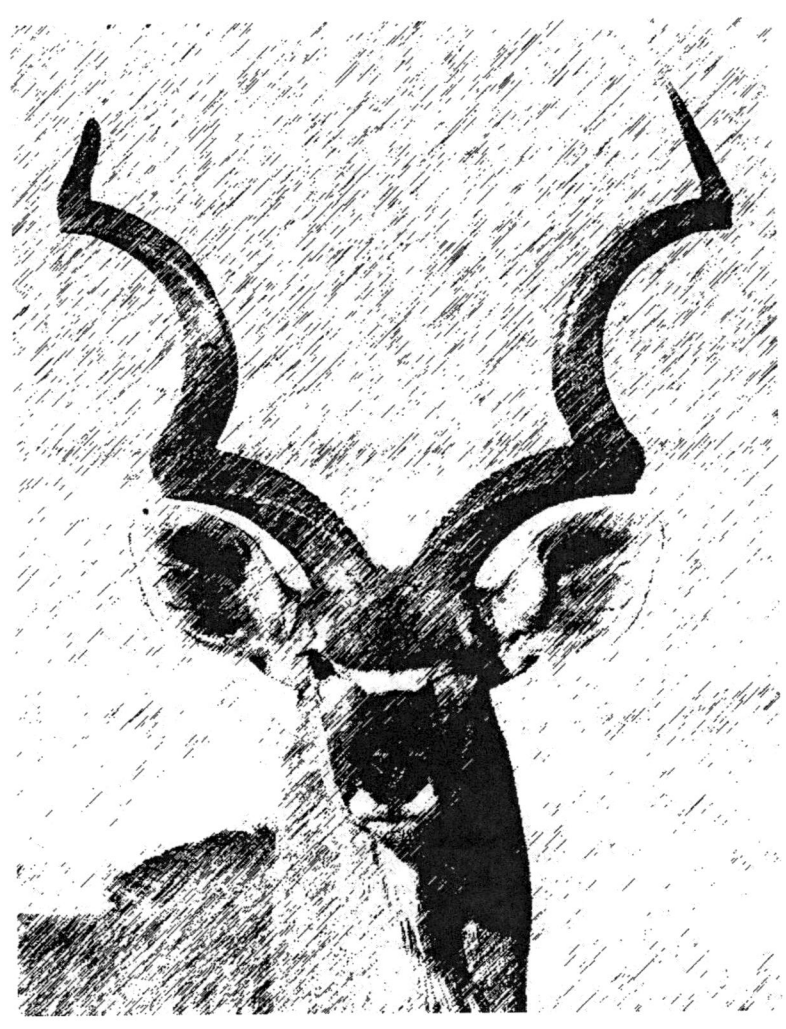

ABOUT THE AUTHOR

Gerard Falotico was 57 at the time he ran his first marathon in 2011. Born in Brooklyn, and the son of an Italian immigrant, he now lives in Saratoga Springs, New York, with his wife Anna. An avid outdoorsman, Jerry has four children and is currently working as a nurse anesthetist. Between age 55 and 56 he encountered a series of medical problems that forced a radical change in his lifestyle and eating habits, losing 85 pounds in one year. At the behest of a friend, he ran his first race, a 5K race on New Year's Eve, and was hooked. Five months later he ran his second race—a marathon. Since then, he has run a total of four marathons, including the Paris Marathon in April 2013, as well as numerous other races.

CPSIA information can be obtained at www.ICGtesting.com
Printed in the USA
BVOW04s0825150214

344906BV00001B/2/P